The Year of Living Doggedly

See 100 colour photos
from the book online
http://doggedly.ca

The Year of Living Doggedly

Published by *Dogged Publications*
printed by *Lightning Source*

ISBN number

978-0-9880375-0-2

THE YEAR OF LIVING DOGGEDLY

Peter Marmorek

for Diana and Rui: my pack

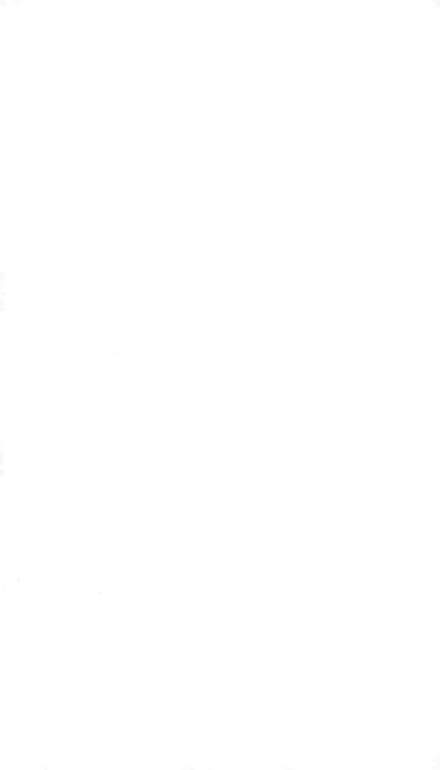

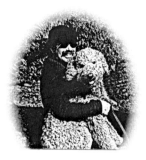

TABLE OF CONTENTS

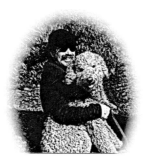

I. Survival of the Cutest

"The whole world reminds me of my dog
My dog reminds me of the whole world."

Jane Siberry, *Everything Reminds Me of my Dog*

In our second week at the rented cottage in Gaspé we set out on a July hike through the woods and up into the mountains, along a path that hid its memory of once having been a road beneath layers of grasses and shrubs. It might still be able to impersonate one well enough to fool a skidoo driver during the seven months Gaspésian winter. Rui was enthusiastically exploring all the strange smells he was picking up, so different from the Toronto scents he'd come to know in the last nine months, and he politely ignored Diana and me as we speculated about him.

We were musing over whether this urban dog could survive on his own, out here in the natural world, whether there was some ecological niche he could squeeze into if we both disappeared, perhaps suddenly sucked up by visiting aliens. I was dubious; neither his frozen reaction to a rabbit crossing the trail, nor his panicked cowering when a grouse flew up in front of him gave any reason to hope he could compete with native coyotes, foxes, or bears whose prey he'd be after, or whose prey he might more likely be. It had been many generations since any of his ancestors, either poodle or Labrador retriever, had lived in the wild and taught hunting skills to their offspring. I was worried about his chances, and thought we'd somehow have to persuade the aliens to take him along.

Diana was smarter.

"He's learned to survive," she observed. "He'd just head back down this road, find some people, and be so charming and adorable they'd take him in."

I laughed; she was right, of course. Dogs survive in this dog-eat-dog world by appealing to humans and knowing how to fill our emotional needs. I suddenly flashed back to a survival course at Queen's University where I had taken my teacher training 35 years earlier. You had to survive a weekend in New York City after being dropped off with nothing but 25¢ in your pocket. One classmate coped by panhandling until he had enough money, then finding out from other street people where the cheap flophouses were, spending the night in one, panhandling some more for food the next day, and eventually getting through the forty-eight hours. Another classmate took his quarter and used it to phone Columbia University's Teacher's College. He explained where he was, told the story of how he came to be there, and after Columbia students came and picked him up, they partied all weekend.

Rui would survive in exactly that way, not by taking care of himself, but by finding people whom he could convince to take care of him. I was reassured; I hadn't felt at all certain about my abilities to meet the communication challenge of convincing the aliens they really wanted a ten month old puppy along.

Later that evening we were all back in the sitting room at the cottage. Diana was knitting a hat for her mother, Brenda, while I tried to solve yet another New York Times crossword. Rui was playing with what was left of a bright yellow squeaky toy, after he'd gnawed off its legs, and killed its squeaker. It was really just a torn hollow rubber ball, but he would squeeze it in his jaws, then let it go, then squeeze it, then drop it, then pounce on it, then squeeze it again for hours. He'd held on to it through the entire walk that day, letting it go only to take a drink when he was crossing a stream. Unlike the kitchen water dish at which he usually drinks, the stream had a lively current which swept the squeaky toy away. Rui furiously chased it and caught it around the second bend. Perhaps he could catch mice in the wilderness, if they squeaked loudly enough and had their legs gnawed off.

That evening he was playing with it next to the mint-green couch I was on. Sometimes he'd bat it across the room and ferociously pursue it, or drop it in front of us so we'd toss it and he could pounce on it. He was absolutely focused on this game, the most enticing part of which seemed to be chewing and batting at the toy while lying down next to the couch. There was a ruffled frill there that covered the six inch gap between the bottom of the upholstery and the floor. That meant the squeaky toy could easily roll under the couch, and it often did. Every time that happened, Rui would try to squirm his head under the couch, so we'd just see his rear end wriggling as he passionately tried to recover his Precious. Sometimes he'd succeed, but often he didn't, and he'd alternate trying to wiggle under the couch with staring mournfully at where the toy had last been seen, making little moaning sounds. Eventually Diana or I would take pity on his desperation, getting out the broom and batting the toy out where he could grab it. I was curious as to why he played with the squeaky next to the couch, the only place in the house where he would keep losing it. Surely he was smart enough to understand that when it rolled under the couch he couldn't get at it, so why did he keep doing that over and over?

Suddenly the penny dropped. Of course he could get at it. He just had to look cute, and Diana or I would retrieve it for him. I remembered Roy, my long ago friend in the late 1960's when we were both at MIT. He was majoring in electrical engineering while I was studying psychology. We were working on modifying the standard issue telephone in my room, so it could connect to three separate phone systems rather than one, could flash silently rather than ring when I needed to sleep at unusual hours, could allow me to put calls on hold, and could patch different calls together. Roy had been teasing me electrical engineering was a more useful major than psychology because it had given him the skills to do those kinds of things, skills I didn't have. I thought about his point, and admitted those were indeed useful skills, but added perhaps psychology was the reason it was in my room that he had wound up using them.

I had been an undergraduate then, but Rui must be working on his graduate degree in owner psychology. Really, why does he need opposable thumbs as long as he can get us to use ours to give him exactly what he wants? I'd been superficially thinking of survival as a prey-predator competition for food. But besides physical needs, humans have emotional needs: to be loved, to give love, to be entertained, to be needed. New breeds like labradoodles are designed to fill those emotional needs, and they will survive and prosper in proportion to how well they do that. For the past nine months I'd been thinking we were training Rui so his behaviour would better fit our preferences, but at the same time he'd been training us just as assiduously to meet his. It was a sobering thought, particularly for a man who was lying on his stomach squirming to reach a yellow squeaky toy that lay just out of his reach under the couch.

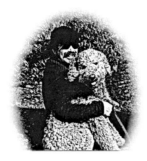

2. The Dog-shaped Hole

"And I just don't know what happens next,
Looks like freedom, but it feels like death,
It's something in between, I guess,
It's closing time"

Leonard Cohen, *Closing Time*

I had known 2005 was some kind of turning point, even when I was in it. Do caterpillars know what they will turn into, as they seal up the cocoon? The previous June I'd stopped teaching high school, after having done that for a third of a century. It felt as though I'd always been a high school teacher, and now I wasn't any more. When someone asks you, "What do you do?" they are really asking what your job is. And for the first time in my life, I didn't have an answer.

So I spent a year exploring that hole in my life, feeling gingerly around the edges of the empty space. Not having a job meant in October and November I was able to more fully support both my father as he bravely faced his death from a failing liver, and my mother as she struggled to find her life without him in a home they'd lived in together for longer than I'd been teaching.

5

In January, I went back to MIT, the place that since the sixties has always felt like my real home, hoping there I'd be re-inspired. January is MIT's "Independent Activities Period", a month of free non-credit courses, on everything from outdoor survival to Turkish film, from quantum string theory to how the brain processes dreams, from the meditative painting of Tibetan tsa–tsas to the finer points of chocolate tasting. I challenged myself to write about every course on my blog, whether about the content, the people, or the experience of being totally lost (string theory fitted there.) One day MIT featured my blog on their homepage, and to my amazement people seemed to really like what I had written. Perhaps I still was a teacher, just not one in high school.

Back in Toronto later that spring, that insight led me to create "The Writers' Croft", an online course in creative writing. I built a website, bought some Google-flavoured publicity, was given some more as a heart gift from a friend, and watched with pleasure as it started to grow. Looking for a community, I joined Tikkun Toronto, a group of mostly Jewish men and women who met every three weeks to heal and repair the world. They welcomed me, and I became their computer guy, running their website and editing a weekly newsletter. Increasingly, I had a lot to do, most of which seemed to involve my sitting alone in front of a computer screen. It was good for my mind, but less good for my body. How I could get back into exercising remained a question I was definitely going to deal with, tomorrow.

Diana, my wife, had been tremendously supportive of my search, and having seen her leave a secure job in collegiate administration a few years earlier for art had given me the confidence to leap into my void. But during the day she was now either teaching art at Humber college, or working in her studio creating it, while I was in our empty house. And neither sitting alone in front of a computer upstairs, nor exercising alone downstairs gave me a community. It surprised me how much I missed the school community, both the teachers and students. There were invitations to department parties, but everyone talked about school, and I wasn't part of that any more. While there was more freedom, and things to keep me busy, I became increasingly aware of the presence of an empty space in my life, even if I couldn't name it or outline its shape.

Over the summer Diana and I decided to take a long postponed trip to England, to see friends and relatives. Our marriage survived both learning to drive the rented car counter-intuitively clockwise around roundabouts and somehow navigating London to find Erin and Julia's house in Brixton, where we'd be staying. We'd expected our two friends there, but there was a third. That was Miss Holly Dog, a (mostly) border collie. A day later Holly had stopped barking at us every time we came in, which meant we were now family. As part of being a good guest, I even dared to try taking her for a walk to the wilds of nearby Brockwell park. It was the first time I'd ever taken a dog for a walk, and I was surprised how easy it was, foolishly assuming this was due to some skill I had, rather than to Miss Holly Dog herself. I obviously didn't yet know how good border collies were at herding sheep.

As we walked through Brixton, I could see how it was becoming gentrified, very different from the unassimilated immigrant area it had been in 1971, when I had taught there. I had been working at the London School of Economics, and was bored silly doing the statistical analysis MIT had trained me for. A friend suggested teaching, because British schools were desperate for Maths teachers. I applied for three positions, (never having either taught or been in a British school) and got three job offers; they were clearly pretty desperate. I chose Stockwell Manor, in Brixton, because it seemed a less battered building than the others and the surreal Dali print in front of the office appealed to me . (I hadn't yet learned to recognize foreshadowing.)

As Miss Holly Dog walked beside me, and sat patiently for traffic lights, I mused on how much easier she was to control than some of my students had been. On day one Hope, a thirteen year old Jamaican girl, stood up at the beginning of the very first class I had ever taught, and asked, "Sir, are you a virgin or not?" Terrified, knowing instantly either "yes" or "no" was a very wrong answer, I brusquely suggested she could ask the head master if she wanted to pursue such questions. She declined, and we went back to math. It took about two years before I figured out the right answer to Hope's question was, "Why is that important to you?" Miss Holly Dog, by contrast, got all the answers she needed through inquisitive sniffing, and no disciplinary threats were needed.

I was amazed, as our United Kingdom and Irish trip went on, how everyone we stayed with had dogs. Everyone loved their dog, and they all seemed friendly and sociable. Perhaps too sociable; even then I could see Mungo and Lupe needed more training. Mungo was a chocolate lab whose energy was disturbingly inexhaustible, and Lupe, a border collie, was the alpha in his family. He sprawled on the couch, while everyone else sat on uncomfortable chairs. But Wolf, suspected to be mostly German Shepherd, was happy to go on long meandering walks with his master across the Irish fields, never straying far away. Unlike Miss Holly Dog, in central London, Wolf didn't even need a leash.

Owning a dog...I imagined coming home, while Diana was away teaching or making art in her studio, and always finding someone there who loved me, for whom I was the most wonderful fantastic being in the universe, who would never complain: who wouldn't want that? A dog would be a wonderful reason to go for long walks and finally get enough exercise. Surely training couldn't be so hard? All I'd have to do was just tell it "No!" in a loud voice a few times and it would learn what not to do.

Success comes, I've always believed, when you leap at a crack that suddenly opens in the wall of possibility, rather than through detailed plans on how to scale the wall. Sometimes the leaps are misguided of course, which helps to explain why I own so much electronic junk bought on sale at really great prices. But a sudden crack was how I had entered teaching, back in Brixton. This year had been spent peering around, waiting for the next crack to open, ready to leap. Now that empty space in my life seemed to coalesce into a dog-like shape. And I was very eager to fill it.

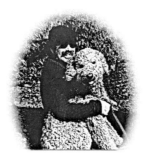

3. ENTER THE RUI BEAST

"...hounds and greyhounds, mongrels, spaniels, curs,
Shoughs, water-rugs and demi-wolves, are clept
All by the name of dogs: the valued file
Distinguishes the swift, the slow, the subtle,
The housekeeper, the hunter, every one
According to the gift which bounteous nature
Hath in him closed"

Macbeth (chatting about dogs to the two murderers)

After the trip was finished, Diana and I returned to our lives in Toronto. I sat in front of the computer and put together weekly issues of my online magazine and tried to come up with supportive and insightful things to say about the work my online students were doing in my writing course. From time to time I would slink past Ahnold, my weight machine, who sat glowering at me in the basement as I tried not to catch his eye. Diana was juggling teaching art at a community college and digital darkroom skills at a photography school, while continuing to work on her own burgeoning art career. It was a busy time.

But the fantasy of a dog stayed with me, and Diana and I occasionally chewed on the idea of becoming dog owners. At first Diana was less enthusiastic than I was. She pointed out that neither of us had ever owned a dog, and that she was running as fast as she could to keep up with her new careers. But I lured her onto the slippery slope with questions such as "Well, just suppose we did get a dog, what kind would we get?" (I had learned this technique when travelling in India, where the carpet salesmen had always been quick to agree they fully understood I was not going to buy a carpet, but they were just curious as to which of their carpets I would buy, if I had been going to buy one. Then they would admire the excellence of my taste, repeat how they knew that I wasn't going to buy any carpet, and ask what I thought would be a fair price for such a fine carpet for someone – certainly not me! – who was going to buy it. And it's a very lovely carpet that I now own, well worth what I overpaid for it.)

So we bought a book listing breeds and their characteristics, carefully eliminating those that said "challenging to train", or "not a beginners' dog." It quickly became clear I envisioned a much bigger dog than Diana did. But there was an intersection point between the biggest canine she was comfortable with and the smallest I was, somewhere around 40 lbs, or 20 kg. We liked the idea of a poodle mix, as we both had allergies and had heard poodle crosses were non-allergenic. And gradually labradoodles, an increasingly popular cross between poodles and Labrador retrievers came to be the breed about which we talked the most. They combined the friendliness and sociability of labs with the non-allergenic, non-shedding coats of poodles, and as poodles come in all sizes, so did labradoodles.

But if we had wanted to buy a labradoodle, were they even available and at what cost? I researched them on the internet, and contacted local breeders, not to buy a dog of course, but just to know what the options were if we did decide to buy a dog in the future. As no one had any pups available we relaxed, as we didn't have any decision to make, and discussed further theoretical questions, such as the putative puppy's name. Diana felt we should call him

Rui, after a local Portuguese politician whose unsuccessful campaign we had both supported a few years earlier. I felt we should wait, and the dog would reveal its name to us in its own time, but as we didn't have a dog and hadn't officially decided to get one, there was no reason to put much energy into debating what to call this non-presence.

On Friday, November 3rd, 2006 things shifted, and that sudden crack opened in the wall. Marguerite, Diana's sister-in-law, was staying with us for the annual Toronto Royal Winter fair. Diana's brother Rowan and Marguerite owned the sheep farm with 750 ewes (the one run by the border collie, Lupe) on which we'd stayed in Scotland during lambing season. She was the secretary of the Scottish Clydesdale society, and the Royal Winter Fair is a Very Big Thing in the world of Clydesdales, who are themselves very big things in the world of horses.

And that was the moment Paddy O'Hare, one of the labradoodle breeders I had contacted, emailed me. An order had just been cancelled. A couple who lived on the 22nd floor of a condo had woken up and realized that wasn't a great place to raise a young puppy and wanted to back out. Paddy attached an insanely cute picture of this puppy who had become available, but warned us a number of other people were also interested, so if we wanted this dog we needed to act fast.

I muttered Rabbi Hillel's saying, "If not now, when?" and talked to Diana. She praised me for how much I had supported her in her new challenges, and said she would support me if I decided to get a dog but I had to agree that the training and nurturing of the puppy would be primarily my task. We discussed the possibility of going to Grand Bend, a three hour drive, to look at the pup. Not to get it, you understand, but just to see it. Marguerite was enthusiastic, not just because she was an animal person, but as it would be a chance for her to see rural Ontario. So as good hosts, how could we say no?

So we drove, stopped in Stratford for lunch where we showed Marguerite the famed Shakespearian theatres, and found an ice arena open for hockey practice, which allowed not only a look at authentic Canadian culture, but accessible washrooms. Then we drove some more, and walked along the chilly shores of Lake Huron and came eventually to Paddy's and saw the pup, who was even cuter in the fur than in pixels. Diana called "Rui" and he wiggled his bum at her, his universal response to all attention. At that moment we knew, (as we had really known in our hearts all along) that we would get him, even though we didn't know anything about looking after young puppies (but we had Marguerite there, for one more day, and she did). And so a nine week old Rui, covered with soft apricot curls, came bounding into our lives. We paid Paddy, who gave us Rui's official papers, a cage, and some photocopied instructions on raising puppies. Then Diana drove the three hours back to Toronto while Rui wriggled happily on my lap, and vomited periodically.

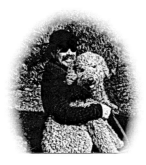

4. WHAT HAVE I DONE?

"Human beings, who are almost unique in having the ability to learn from the experience of others, are also remarkable for their apparent disinclination to do so."

Douglas Adams, *Last Chance to See*

I wondered how many new parents there were who came home with their new baby and felt as we did, that they had casually drifted into an incredibly dumb decision that would utterly destroy their previously happy lives for the foreseeable future? The first night we tried having Rui sleep in our bedroom in a puppy-sized cage Paddy had given us, and he moaned and whined for half an hour before falling to sleep. Then in the middle of the night Diana got up, and he started moaning again. She took him outside (which he liked). But clearly being put back in his cage was an unhappy experience, so he moaned and struggled till it became just as unhappy for us too. It all seemed a bit overwhelming, and his throwing up on the carpet in the computer room added to the stress...none of us got much sleep that night.

I kept remembering the Cyclone, a rickety wooden roller-coaster I once rode at Coney Island and the feeling on that first long climb up when it really sank in that I couldn't get off and was irrevocably committed. When the coaster took off I'd hung on and grasped the rail in front of me trying to see what would happen next, and how to get through it. And somewhere in the back of my mind was the knowledge this was all supposed to be fun. I consoled myself about Rui by remembering how amidst the Cyclone terror, I realized I really was enjoying some parts of the ride after all. I just needed to hang on through the first turns and twists, and the good parts would come.

The next day we sleepily said goodbye to Marguerite, who was flying back to Scotland, and she wished us luck with Rui and assured us everything would work out just fine. Easy for her to say…she was escaping, while we were left to deal with the increasingly obvious problem that Rui was not as housebroken as he had been said to be at Paddy's. Perhaps he was housebroken, but only at Paddy's, and he figured our home was a legitimate target. The second night we kept him in the kitchen, but not in his cage. He pooped on the floor, which wasn't surprising, but then pooped in the front hall after being taken for an elimination walk outside, which was depressing. I remembered Kurt Vonnegut reporting his sister wrote after her first baby was born, "Here I am, cleaning shit off practically everything". I was beginning to feel like that.

We left Rui trapped behind closed kitchen doors while I fled to our nearest Pet Valu store to shop for toys, leashes, nail clippers, and doggy treats. I often avoided dealing with threats from the unknown by buying things, in the hope that if I gave burnt offerings to the God of Commerce, He'd intervene in the cosmos on my behalf. I found on return that Rui had held off until he was outside, which might have been a sign my sacrifice had been deemed acceptable. I hastily browsed Amazon, which allowed me to make further one-click sacrifices, ordering the first of an increasingly large number of books I would accumulate on how to raise puppies. I wrote to Paddy hoping for clues, and he was supportive but without the magical answer I wanted.

Rui had peed on the floors twice, so we were pleased that when he had arrived we had quickly taken up all the carpets (including my favourite from India). He also really liked chewing anything, from the honeysuckle vine we had hoped would someday cover our backyard trellis, to all the electric and stereo wiring which snake along our floorboards. The wires were dangerous; I knew I'd forever feel an utter failure if I electrocuted my new puppy within a week of getting him, so I raced to Ikea and bought Tubli, which was a clever set of plastic tubes which snapped around electric wires either to protect them (which was my theory) or to serve as warm-up chewing practice (which was Rui's).

But the biggest crisis seemed to be that I had blithely ignored Wikipedia's warning that while labradoodles are significantly better than most dogs in terms of causing allergies, they aren't universally non-allergenic, and the degree varies unpredictably, even within a single litter. Two days after getting Rui, both of us suddenly developed headaches, Diana with wheezing and shortness of breath as well. I could hardly bear to think of what that meant, as we tried to cope both with a wild puppy, and our physical reactions. I wrote in my journal "Yesterday morning Diana and I confessed to each other that we both felt like crying. And what makes it so hard is that clearly none of this is in any way Rui's fault...he's being a puppy, playful and wild, just as he should be. And that makes me feel worse...it's our fault, we're not able to cope. I like him more and more, but we can't face fifteen years of headaches, and breathing is one of those essential functions. He's lying at my feet looking up at me as I write this, and my head is throbbing painfully, and the tears are rolling down my cheeks, and I just hope that someday Rui and I can laugh about all this."

That evening I went in to pick up our 11 year old nephew, Sam, at his school. Diana had looked after him for one day a week since his birth, and he and I had become increasingly and joyfully closer in the ten years that Diana and I had been together. Sam's moms had strongly supported Diana and me getting a dog as Sam had been talking about getting one. They thought this would be a fine way for him to learn what was involved without their having to commit. I drove up to his school, and as I walked into the classroom, his teacher looked up blearily, and moaned about how everyone at the school had a headache and allergy-like reactions, and wasn't this autumn weather terrible? She seemed a bit taken aback when I responded, "You have a bad headache? That's wonderful news!" That night Toronto had a thunderstorm, the weather system shifted, and no allergic reactions to Rui have ever been reported again. We were through our first bout of post–puppy depression.

Looking after a puppy, I rapidly learnt, seemed to be a full time job, which was hard, as I had a few other jobs that had to be put on hold, or postponed altogether, because puppies – or at least Rui – turned out to be quite talented at getting into trouble, or at getting your attention by chewing on you, or anything they else can get at. It wasn't as bad as owning two parrots (two brave and crazy friends I've had did that, and the birds happily chewed through whatever they could get to, which – as they could fly – was absolutely everything there was.) I supposed a monkey would be even worse, but I wasn't eager to find out, except anecdotally. Again I thought of new parents I knew who had planned to have both parents return to work quickly and found that impossible. I consoled myself by remembering how they all said (much later) it was the best decision they had ever made. And everyone told me Rui should be house-trained faster than a baby.

He instantly took to sitting on my lap and — as Wikipedia predicted— he enjoyed water: baths were a pleasure. I really liked this: Gummitch, a brilliant and irascible cat with whom I once lived, used to consider herself defeated if she emerged from a bath without having drawn a quantity of blood greater than the amount of water in the tub. Often, she wasn't defeated. Rui simply lay down in warm water and enjoyed it.

He was certainly able to learn things, figuring out in two days how the front and back stairs work and climbing up and down happily. Then he figured out how to leap onto the couch, and I started the process of convincing him that this was a taboo. He started the process of convincing me that I really wanted to have him with me there. For a while it would be unclear who was the more convincing. His big step forward on the third day was going for a walk on a leash. When I first put it on him in the backyard he decided this was a fish-escapes-lure kind of game, and leapt around enthusiastically, chewed on the leash and tugged as vigorously as a four kilogram puppy could. But when I got him onto the sidewalk he trotted happily along beside me, with occasional tangles, but clearly willing to let me lead him (as long as he could stop and sniff from time to time at all these exciting new smells.)

He met a German shepherd about three times his size (though only a month older) and while the two sniffed at each other, I talked to the dog's owner and realized how easy it was to chat with other people about their animals. I'd lived in the neighbourhood for over twenty-five years, the German Shepherd's owner lived just down the block, yet I had no memory of ever having noticed him before. I suddenly realized that there was a whole world out there of people who loved to talk about their dogs , and I had the entry card to that world, right at the end of my leash. Then we ran back home; Rui and I were able to run at about the same speed at this point and we both enjoyed it. His first walk was at least a half mile and I rewarded him with a Pet-Valu recommended freeze-dried liver treat, which he went crazy for, and after which he licked me all over, hoping to find more.

Rui would come when he was called (some of the time) and responded to "NO!" He didn't always stop whatever he was doing, but sometimes he did. I thought he seemed to know that he should stop, but I might have been projecting here. The best way to communicate displeasure seemed to be to growl; he either stopped what he was doing, or rolled over onto his back. My start at reading puppy manuals lead me to understand he was acknowledging that I was the top dog, which was certainly my theory about how this was going to work. I knew positive reinforcement was supposed to be better than negative, but it was when he started doing something wrong (peeing on the floor, chewing on the couch) that I most strongly reacted. That was sadly similar to teaching: when my students were working I didn't say anything until I noticed that they were sending emails to a friend, or doing math homework.

I didn't really feel as though I'd started training him yet, but I remembered once reading that all television was educational; the only question was what it was teaching. So perhaps everything I did with Rui was training. I was happy that I was managing to live with him, and nothing terrible had happened to either of us. By the end of the first week he had started to learn house-training, which came as a huge relief, both to us and the house floors. Still, it felt a bit like wandering through a maze with my eyes closed. All right, so far.

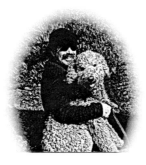

5. My Non-Pet History

"I meant what I said, and I said what I meant.
And an elephant's faithful, one hundred percent."

Dr. Seuss, *Horton Hatches the Egg*

Neither my brother David nor I had pets when we were growing up in the 1950's. I only know through my parents telling the story that when I was three they bought me a goldfish. But they kept it in its original small bowl without aeration and it died fairly soon as a result. Worried that I would be traumatized by its death, they swiftly replaced it with an identical specimen. But soon it too swam after its predecessor to that more oxygenated goldfish bowl in the sky. After the third goldfish had equally quickly shuffled off its mortal scale, my parents decided I was old enough to learn about death. I appeared to cope, or so they tell me. I have no memory of the incident, but I can't decide whether that's because of deep repression, poor memory or the intrinsic boringness of goldfish. At no point during ten later years of therapy did any of the goldfish ever surface, even floating belly up. But those three dead fish were as close to pets as I would get in my childhood.

I almost had a second pet: a one inch long green turtle I spotted crawling in the gutter outside our house in Granby, a small French-Canadian town in Quebec's Eastern Townships. The Granby lake was six blocks away, and I immediately understood, with the certainty of childhood, that the turtle had obviously crawled that far to find me. I was eight years old, but already I recognized such a heroic quest should be rewarded. I got out a large glass bowl, created a sandy island surrounded by water, finally adding the turtle and some lettuce. The turtle was indifferent to the lettuce, but became enthusiastic when I added some small bits of the fresh liver Mom had been planning to serve us for dinner that evening. It stared fixedly at the morsels, then lunged and devoured them in voracious bites. I was deeply impressed, as I'd never managed to develop the slightest degree of comparable enthusiasm for liver, despite persistent parental encouragement. I immediately understood how this turtle might be very useful to me and asked my mother if I could keep it as a pet.

My mother, a German banker's daughter, had been raised with a well-founded fear of signing blank checks so we went the next day to Granby's only pet store to learn more about the turtle. The young man behind the counter examined it, and explained this was a snapping turtle which eventually would grow to over two feet in length and weigh over forty pounds. I was enraptured; visions of a perfectly trained killer turtle flashed though my mind. "Thunderer: attack!" I would order, and Thunderer would lurch Golem-like toward my enemies as though they were no more than tiny pieces of liver. Sadly, my parents were clear, unambiguous, and united that a snapping turtle had no place in their vision of whom I was going to become, and Thunderer was released back onto the shores of Granby lake, where he probably lived out his sad and lonely life, haunted forever by memories of fresh raw liver.

Slightly earlier there had been Ambika, my Indian elephant. She entered my life on an otherwise uneventful day in 1952 when my father was reading *Le Voix de l'Est* (The Voice of the East) our local

French daily. I was five, so Dad read out an article to me, translating into English as he went. The article quoted Prime Minister Nehru of the then newly formed country of India saying that if "the children of Granby wanted an elephant for the zoo, he would try to dig one up." Our mayor had just founded the Granby Zoo, and had travelled to India to solicit contributions, so I suspect Nehru was looking for good publicity in Commonwealth countries for his new state. But back in 1952, all I heard was the offer of a free elephant. I was sure I knew everything about them, as one of my favourite books was Dr. Seuss' story of how heroic Horton the elephant had sat in a tree for months to hatch the egg of Mayzie the lazy bird. I jumped to my feet and said, "Can I write to him?"

Dad typed my letter from dictation, which included my observing that, "I didn't know elephants lived underground." (I was puzzled by the "digging up" part of Nehru's offer.) It turned out that there was an attempt to coordinate a collective letter from Granby's French school children, but long before their letter got organized, (ah, early intimations of educational bureaucracy!) I had received a letter back from Nehru, with the official seal of India in red sealing wax, explaining that he would send me an elephant which, he added, was a large creature that did not live underground, but roamed through forests. Worthy of note were his hand-written grammatical corrections on the letter, and that the answer was received two weeks after we had mailed the original letter. Dad and Mom notified the Mayor of Granby; he notified the press; I became an instant celebrity.

The story spread across Canada, and through the north-eastern US, as far west as Chicago and as far south as New York. It was my first lesson in media distortion; in the news stories my age ranged from five to twelve, sometimes there were two elephants, other times the elephant had already arrived. My parents decided appearing on national TV was not what I needed, so I missed out on that. But it was still very heady stuff, culminating two years later when the four year old Ambika arrived in Granby complete with her mahout to help her initiation into this land of snow. I had to officially present her to the zoo, and made my speech. I was relaxed about the speech part, but nervous about standing next to Ambika; even though she was three years younger than me, she easily outweighed me by a factor of ten. My parents reassuringly explained that elephants were vegetarian, and only ate vegetables. I thought about this and then asked, "But how does the elephant know that I'm not a vegetable?" Maybe she didn't and just wasn't hungry but she seemed very friendly, and I still have the photos of us in the family's official elephant album.

Time passed, and while I visited Ambika often, I didn't really think she knew who I was, or that it was my fault she wound up in small town Quebec. Then I moved to Montreal, on to Toronto; life happened, and I lost touch with her. I did get to travel through India, and I suspect that part of its draw lay in Ambika from whom I had learned that country was a magical place; if you wrote to it, they would send you an elephant. On my first day in Delhi, jet-lagged after an overnight flight from Cairo, I forgot that Indian traffic moves on the left side of the road. I looked the wrong way, and woke up to a shout from the mahout riding a large and much painted elephant parading through the Chandi Chowk, the old market in which I was staying. Never have I escaped a near fatal traffic accident with such delight – India was a country in which you could get stepped on by an elephant. It was instant love.

Years later I would be teaching linear equations to a restive Grade 9 Math class at Clarkson. There were a few minutes left before the bell, so I told them the elephant story. One of the students, Nadia, who had just come to our school from Madras, India, got very excited. She blurted to the class that when she'd been studying Indian history at home, their history books had told how Nehru had sent an elephant to a small boy in Canada. And here the small boy was, all grown up and teaching her linear equations. My fifteen minutes of fame had been immortalized; I had made it into the history books. But while I deeply admired Ambika, she was never really a personal pet.

Occasionally the family talked about getting a dog or a cat. But both my parents worked, and while Mom had grown up with dogs, she didn't want to look after them, and suspected that neither my brother David nor I would be reliable enough that she wouldn't have to. So it wasn't until I was 25, married to Jan, and living in Cobalt, that I got my first real pet. I was a second year English teacher in a remote town in Northern Ontario, and Jan had grown up with pets, so we thought a kitten would be easy to manage, and found Gummitch. She was black, with a white spot at her throat. I was impressed with her at the pet store because she was the most active, running enthusiastically around her cage and meowing constantly. I took these as appealing features, a perspective I would later come to regret. Perhaps the meowing seemed less conspicuous next to the African Grey parrot in the store, which performed a splendid and impeccable imitation of the cough of a dying man who had smoked three packs of cigarettes a day for fifty years. The parrot interrupted this continual coughing only to let loose a 135 decibel wolf whistle, after which it would cackle quietly to itself and go back to coughing. Parrots live for a long time, and this one may still be there, waiting for someone crazy enough to want to live with its repertoire.

Gummitch's name came from a great Fritz Lieber short story, the opening line of which was, "Gummitch was a super-kitten, with an IQ of 178." Our Gummitch did show her intelligence in a number of ways, most of them antisocial. She quickly learned that we would not always get her food when she went to the fridge and meowed, but we would let her outside when she went to the front door and did the same. So she would go to the door, meow, and then when either Jan or I would arrive, she'd run over to the fridge.

Gummitch had an intuitive understanding of political protest, as I suspect many cats do. When I left her with my parents while Jan and I were away on a trip, she didn't like that, and engaged in what my mother delicately called, "protest movements", leaving small offerings all around the house. At one point, I got the idea of walking her on a leash, after seeing a neighbour doing that with his cat. (In retrospect, it was probably a small dog dressed in a cat costume for Halloween.) When I finally won a savage fight and got the harness on, Gummitch immediately fell over and lay motionless on the floor. I panicked. Had I broken some bone? I tore the harness off, and Gummitch leapt to her feet, miraculously healed. I sighed, and put the harness on her again. She fell over and lay still again. I dragged her around our apartment, but she would not move. I carefully felt around the harness which was suitably loose, not constricting her. But while it was on she simply wouldn't move. As soon as it was removed, Gummitch was back to normal. No cooperation with evil; Ghandi would have been proud of her.

But unlike Ghandi, she was not non-violent. She hated everyone except Jan and me, and was never completely sure about Jan. She would happily claw anyone else, given a chance. Her one social skill was her ability to catch hard cat food in the air when I tossed it to her; her record, I still remember, was 17 in a row. And she loved our water bed, and never attacked it with her claws, though she would stand amazed for hours, pushing down a spot, then watching it come back to its original level.

But I loved her, and was heartbroken when my body reacted to our move to Toronto by developing a severe allergy to cats. For a year I got shots once a week to try and persuade my body to tolerate them, but when I wound up in hospital on IV after a severe asthma attack, it was clear that either Gummitch or I had to leave. Jan and I found a farm that took her in, and the only pet I ever had was gone. I missed her, but I couldn't live with a cat. At that time it seemed as though a dog would be too much work; I didn't understand how with the right dog that work could become pleasure.

Later, when I was married to Cath, I shared a house with Wicca, a cockatiel. He was not intelligent, even by cockatiel standards, which are fairly low, and living with him led me to understand why "bird-brain" is so rarely a compliment. But he did understand

and seek attention: if Cath and I were playing Scrabble, he would land on the Scrabble board and peck savagely at the tiles until we paid attention to him.

But he was not my pet. Wicca was Cath's pet, and it became very clear that as far as he was concerned, I was a rival up with whom he would not put. To him, I was no more than a larger and more irritating Scrabble tile. He would attack me viciously whenever he was out of the cage, which Cath found very amusing. I would wipe off the blood and smile weakly.

So I confess to being less heartbroken than Cath on the day Wicca flew the coop. We tried to find him and even ran ads, but when we drove to see the lost and found cockatiels it was immediately clear none was Wicca. Not by their looks (cockatiels only have about three styles of feathers, and these looked pretty similar even to Cath) but by their behaviour. These cockatiels allowed me to pet them without even trying to peck me. It was clear they weren't Wicca, who was never heard of again.

And since then there had been no pet in the house. The years passed, Cath and I first separated and then divorced, and eventually Diana and I came to live together. We created a water feature in our Toronto back yard, then stocked it with some goldfish who ate mosquito larvae in the summer, stayed in the aquarium of a friend in Oakville, (Canada's richest suburb!) in the winter, and didn't die. There was a rat who lived in the compost at the end of the garden and had her children there, and a raccoon who bedded down in the empty computer boxes stored in the garage until I installed a motion-sensitive shrieking white plastic skull (Yorick) that drove him away. But none of these were really personal relationships, except possibly poor Yorick, whom (alas!) I knew well.

Yorick required no training. I turned him on or off, and I fed him new batteries when he stopped shrieking, which is just the opposite of pets one feeds when they start shrieking. The goldfish would come to the surface when I sprinkled food on it, but that surface was really the only common plane between their world underwater and mine above. But these were all regular duties, not an interaction between owner and pet. Even Gummitch didn't really get trained; we fed her and allowed her to go out and come in. There was nothing in my past that could have given me any clues just how involving and life changing living with a dog would be.

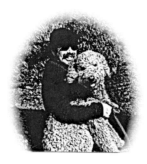

6. Training a Dog

"When I was young
It seemed that life was so wonderful
A miracle, oh it was beautiful, magical
And all the birds in the trees
Well they'd be singing so happily
Joyfully, playfully watching me.
But then they send me away
To teach me how to be sensible
Logical, responsible, practical
And then they showed me a world
Where I could be so dependable...."

Supertramp *The Logical Song*

Back when our conversations about living with a dog were still being conducted in the future conditional tense, Diana and I had agreed that if we were to have one, we would want it to be really well-trained. We'd both been around dogs who leapt up on guests arriving at the door, who nipped at your fingers, who had to be told "No!" over and over again. I had always secretly felt that the owners could have made more of an effort, that really it was their fault and not their dog's. We certainly didn't want a dog like that, and part of the incentive for getting a puppy from a known breeder (as opposed to an unknown rescue dog from a shelter) was to avoid an animal that had been traumatized by its earlier experiences. We wanted a perfect blank page on which to write our masterpiece.

So we bought Rui, knowing that as labradoodles had first been bred to be seeing-eye guide dogs for people with allergies, they were clearly intelligent and capable of being impeccably trained. The key problem was that neither Diana nor I had ever trained a puppy or even lived with one, which made the situation roughly equivalent to buying a large pile of high quality lumber because you've read beautiful houses can be built with it. Intent and materials may be two sides of a triangle, but technique is the third. We had the puppy, and we had the owners, but now what were we supposed to do?

I was home all day with the pup, and I was supposed be the primary trainer. While Rui was innately affectionate and enthusiastic, he wasn't completely housebroken. He liked to nip at my fingers, dressing-gowns, electric wires, or pretty much anything else. We moved wires out of reach and child-proofed the cleaning items cabinet. I came outside and found him by the backyard pond gnawing on a piece of shale about twice his size, possibly working on sharpening his already needle-like teeth. These seemed the sorts of behaviours a trainer should address, but how to begin? Paddy had given us some suggestions in the photocopied binder that came with Rui, including the American Kennel Club's description of the ten behaviours of a "Good Canine Citizen", all of which seemed eminently desirable. Who wouldn't want a dog to "Sit, lie down, and stay on command"? So we were clear on our goals, but foggy on the direction to take us there. Remembering a fine dictum passed on to me by my Uncle Walter, "Time spent on reconnaissance is never wasted," I immediately started researching what to do next.

Google of course led me to thousands of dog-training websites. There were a few points of universal agreement: pushing your pup's nose into his pee, and saying "Bad Dog!" loudly is really ineffective. That eliminated one of the very few things I had thought I knew about dog training. But I did know about teaching teenagers, so I thought about that. What seemed relevant was that my most idyllic years had been in an alternative high school in which each of my students had worked with me one-to-one. A course was completed when all the work was done, whether that took three months, or two years, and the syllabus of each course was shaped by the student and the teacher working together. IndEC had left me a firm believer in individualized education, so I decided not to go to a local dog training school, and instead found a trainer who also believed in the one-to-one method. And so a few weeks later Rui, Diana, and I sat down with Suzanne.

"Magic worker" is not really the right term, because as Arthur Clarke famously wrote, "Any sufficiently advanced technology is indistinguishable from magic". Suzanne knew how to train dogs (or more accurately, how to train their owners) and so while it may have looked like a miracle, the techniques were simple enough that we were able to learn and apply them. We all went to the living room, and then Suzanne led Rui to the kitchen by his leash, said "Kitchen. Wait", and walked away. Rui followed her back into the living room.

She walked him out, firmly, and repeated, "Kitchen. Wait." After about twenty repetitions, he sighed, and lay down there. We tried it next, and it worked again. The next day I tried it and it took about 30 repetitions; Rui wasn't as convinced by me. (I told you he was smart.) But the next time it took three repetitions. Four days later, I told Rui to wait and he waited for one hour in the kitchen while the eight people in my writing group sat in the living room, ten yards away, visible through an open door, and laughed and read and were exactly the sort of people I knew he really wanted to be around. But he waited in the kitchen, occasionally whimpering, but utterly obedient. And he was only eleven weeks old. My guests were amazed, as was I.

So this stuff worked. And that was what was so interesting, because it was a form of teaching — authoritarian, teacher–centred, rigid — that I really hated as a teacher. When Suzanne introduced the concept of boundaries, she said to Diana and me, "You both have to work in your lives, so it's only fair that Rui has to work too. And now we're going to make him work." We both winced. I didn't have to work, and I didn't think anyone else should, let alone an eleven week old puppy. After Suzanne had left, Diana looked at him, and said, "He looks subdued." And it was true, he did.

I went over and looked into his eyes, and gently explained to him that I was the dude, and he was the sub-dude, and that was how it was. The dog training manuals I had looked at had all warned me dogs have a wolf pack mentality and if my dog thought he was the alpha-male in the house, I was going to be very unhappy. I believed he had to be the sub-dude.

And yet... here's a section from the article Suzanne left us on house-breaking (not housetraining, but housebreaking!) *Take him out for one minute maximum, then take him in for 30 minutes, then take him out again. What he has to learn is that he is out for a reason, not just to play around. Let him wait. The longer he waits, the more he will really have to go when he gets to his spot. If, in the process of housebreaking, you miss a few walks, so be it, sometimes life just isn't fair. Besides, there will be times when you just won't be able to take him for a walk, so he might as well get used to your schedule and stop taking so many privileges for granted.*

It did seem a very behaviourist right-wing view; privileges weren't to be taken for granted; they had to be earned. Life wasn't fair, so suck it up and get used to it. Under the new regime, even the dogs will pee on time. All of this made me think about the complex issue of dog's rights. Clearly there was a wide range of answers ranging from PETA to the local K9 Corps. I believed Rui would be happier if he learned to follow the rules we wanted him to follow, and therefore wasn't constantly being reprimanded, but was that just a fascist rationalization? It sounded like a dictatorship warning you that as you'd be happier not to be in prison, don't ever colour outside their lines. What did it say to me about the shallowness of my left-wing political·views if the only way I could train my pup was through right-wing models of conditional love and anal-compulsive toilet training?

I didn't know that answer. I saw how Suzanne seemed to really know how to get Rui to be the well-behaved dog we wanted him to be, and I sure didn't have any better routes for getting there than the ones she was teaching us. I started teaching the way my teachers in high school had taught me: from a position of authority and power. I remembered one of my early mentors, a maths teacher in London, pointing out every teacher's challenge was to find the way that worked for whom they were. She was right. Even though she was a great teacher I couldn't be a great teacher the same way she was; I had to find my own way.

At this point I didn't know dogs in general or Rui specifically enough to have any sense of what would make him happiest, let alone how to balance his happiness against ours. He'd probably have been really happy with sirloin three times a day, which I knew just wasn't going to happen. Chicken kibble was all he got, but with some yogurt on the side, and maybe some ground hamburger from time to time. Good bosses have always known even the sub-dudes deserved some treats.

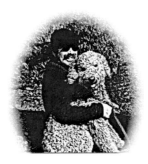

7. The Beast Within

"The beast in me
Is caged by frail and fragile bonds
Restless by day
And by night, rants and rages at the stars
God help, the beast in me"

Nick Lowe, *The Beast in Me*

While I'd imagined dog walks would exercise my legs, Rui was turning out to be at least as much work for my arms. He pulled on the leash about three-quarters of the time, desperately eager to investigate absolutely everything we passed. And while he weighed only seven kilograms at three months which was a lot less than me, I could see that these tug-of-war walks weren't the behaviour we wanted him to develop. And then things went bad.

Suddenly on a Thursday, and again on Friday, Rui became savage at the park. He tore at the leash, barking aggressively, and leapt at my hands, snapping with what seemed like intent to bite. In response, I fastened his leash to a post, walked out of range, and gave him a time out. Then I released him until he snapped again, and so on. For the first time I was really worried; this sort of behaviour in a full grown dog would be dangerously unacceptable. At home, he started snapping at both Diana and I, when we were cuddling him. What had happened to the sweet puppy we had? What had I done wrong? Sudden memories surged of Red Wull, the evil dog who became a ruthless sheep-killer in a nineteenth century book from my childhood. Was Rui a Bad Dog who would grow up to be a sheep-killer, or worse? And that was the lesser of the problems.

The bigger problem was my response. I became furious, yelling at him to stop, dragging him to the pole while screaming, "If you do that again, I'll kill you, you little fucker!" A young puppy can be excused for his poor behaviour; he's learning how the world works, and trying out different strategies. But an adult male in his late 50s? Should be more self-control there, I thought. Except it wasn't about self-control of course, it was about where the anger came from, and why. If I weren't angry, I wouldn't need self-control. I knew I had always gotten angriest when I'd felt I wasn't being seen, when I felt as though I was being ignored. That anger had never proved terribly helpful when dealing with school administration, or misbehaving students, so why would it be with a three month old puppy?

One factor in my choice not to have children was my fear of that anger and rage within me. Perhaps its source lay in a childhood with corporal punishment for infractions such as talking back to my parents, or not doing my homework. As a novice teacher I had cultivated a bad temper, which I had seen as an essential part of the profession. My high school teachers had yelled at me, (and others) so I believed it was a useful way to enforce good behaviour. But in my fourth year of teaching Arlene had come up to me at the end of a class and said, "Sir, you shouldn't yell at us like that." I asked why, feeling a certain righteous sense of thunder-god power which quickly dissipated when she answered, "Because it's so hard to keep from laughing when you do."

After that I had consciously worked to find ways to solve class-room problems other than with verbal violence and by the end of my high school career, homophobia was about the only thing that would instantly push my anger button. But I had always known that my internal volcano was dormant, not extinct, and there was something about living with Rui that was causing eruptions. Getting so angry at a three month old puppy seemed very depressing, so I dealt with it by becoming very depressed.

Fortunately there was a light somewhere in this dark tunnel, and that was our second appointment with Suzanne. We met at 10 on Saturday, and I explained Rui's behaviour and my reactions, but didn't go into huge detail about how badly I felt over not being as calm and consistent an owner as all the books agreed I should be. She suggested taking Rui for a walk, and she'd observe what was happening.

So I did, and she did. He was pulling in all directions, but not barking or snapping. I joked that he was behaving pretty well because she was there, and she said in a certain note of incredulity, "You call that behaving well?" I felt both abashed and cheered: clearly better behaviour was possible.

Then she walked him. In ten minutes he was heeling, staying behind her on the left side, and sitting down when she stopped. And he did the same when I walked him. The keys seemed to be holding the leash more loosely, so that there was no tension for him to pull against, and immediately turning sharply and walking in the opposite direction if he overtook me. As Suzanne said, "You just do the opposite of what he tries to do." It meant we didn't get as far on our walks, but they became much more pleasant.

For the next two days when Rui and I went for walks, things went pretty well. He got snappy after about a half hour when it became clear we weren't going to the park (this constant turning around means a walk becomes much more a process than a destination) but he calmed down as we got home. And when he snapped at me later, I put him in his crate with the door open and made him wait there, which he was very unhappy about just as Suzanne had said he would be. Given the increasing signs of Rui's intelligence, I wondered how long it would be until he figured out that by proper timing of non-heeling, and making me reverse, he could prolong a walk forever; all he'd have to do was just move ahead of me whenever we got close to the house, and I'd head away from it.

But two days later I tried to go for a walk, and Rui kept snapping at the leash, trying to bite it. Each time I would cut things short and bring him home. After four tries, we were both in a state. He ran around the house, refusing to come when I called him, and I finally grabbed him as he tried to dash past me, and stuffed him into his crate. There, he whined piteously and I felt even worse. But when I let him out, he immediately snapped at me, so I put him back. I kept remembering the saying, "Put a liberal up against the wall, and you get a conservative."

It felt like a question of whether I believed in Rousseau's "Noble Savage", or Hobbes' "nasty, coarse, brutish and short". Part of me felt as though I had been given this perfect natural creature, and caused him to become bad by not just letting him be his natural self. Part of me felt if I didn't set absolute rules (no biting, no jumping up) and enforce them with immediate consequences he'd always behave badly. Part of me felt there was something in Rui that caused this, while another was sure the whole situation was my fault. And both images had elements of truth, both for Rui and for me. Both of us were loving creatures, and we needed to learn our boundaries, what we could and couldn't expect from each other.

Part of me felt I'd made a terrible mistake in getting a dog whom I couldn't train properly, and it had all gone pear-shaped, while part of me trusted I just needed to follow the guidelines I'd been given and everything would work out fine. It was probably fair to say that all of me was pretty uncertain about what was happening.

My brother suggested I consider Rui my anger management trainer, and at times when Rui was sleeping peacefully, that was an amusing and insightful way to think of it. But holding on to the distance needed to see that in the heat of a fight was another question. I hoped that just as Suzanne taught me ways to get Rui to behave sedately and maturely, I could learn to do the same. After all, how much less trainable than a three month puppy could this old dog be?

Diana and I noticed part of why Rui was sometimes over the top was simply that he had too much energy. So when he'd been good, we let him run loose in the back yard, which he loved. Because it was December the ground was hard enough that he couldn't dig in the flower beds, so it was a good time to play outside. Rui and I developed a game in which we took turns chasing each other around the yard. We followed this with a second game in which I stood still, panted heavily, and tried to get my breath back while Rui tried to get me to chase him.

Over the next week, I worked consistently with Suzanne's instructions to turn around and walk in the opposite direction when Rui didn't heel. He seemed to be getting more trained, which meant I went off the rails less. I found what worked best when he threw a puppy tantrum was to crouch down, hold him gently but firmly, and talk to him in a calm voice. (This worked well for both of us, in fact.) Dogs instantly pick up very quickly on human moods; there wasn't much hope of fooling him that I was happy when I really was angry.

At the end of that week, Rui had been out in the yard for awhile, and Diana and I went out together to walk him. Part of this was to demonstrate to Diana what Suzanne had been teaching Rui and me, part was for the pleasure of the sunny day and our little community. Rui was wonderfully behaved, not snapping at the leash, but trotting along between us with that lovely high-stepping gait that came from the poodle in his genes. As we walked north up the alleyway behind our house, the sun was directly behind us, and there was a lovely image of our three shadows in front, with Rui's tail wagging happily back and forth as we made our way. It felt as though we were a whole pack, out together. And since for a while the leash biting and leaping problems were over, I could fool myself into thinking my anger issues were over too.

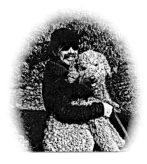

8. Labradoodles and Projection

Now I can understand your tears and your shame.
She called you "boy" instead of your name.
When she wouldn't let you inside.
When she turned and said
"But honey, he's not our kind."

Janis Ian, *Society's Child*

By late fall Rui had gotten his three month round of vaccinations, which allowed him to play with other dogs. He was interested in every dog he met, and even riding in the hatchback of our Toyota Echo, he'd stare out the window in fixated fascination whenever he spotted a dog out in the world. Since he clearly couldn't smell or hear them from inside the car, Diana and I were surprised how clearly he could distinguish between those things that were dogs and the rest of the world. Given that the range of dog sizes and breeds was greater than any other animal, how did he know that a Great Dane and a chihuahua were somehow like him, and a pussycat wasn't? But while Rui didn't distinguish between breeds of dogs, others did. And most curiously, they weren't even dogs.

37

Walking Rui one day, I met my first dog racist. She owned a pure-bred white standard poodle, Molly, who was beautifully coiffed and groomed in that traditional poodle way. Molly was straining at her leash, barking and trying to leap on Rui in exactly the same way Rui tries to leap on dogs he wants to play with. Her owner called her back into a sit, and said, "Molly doesn't like crossbreeds. She only plays with real poodles".

I smiled, feeling incredulous, and responded, "Sounds to me as though there might be some projection going on there."

"Oh no," said Ms. Molly, "I don't think Molly's projecting anything."

And since there was clearly nothing more perfect that could be said, Rui and I wandered off.

Rui is a labradoodle, a descendent of poodles and Labrador retrievers. When Diana and I were debating what kind of dog to get, we talked to friends who had dogs, some of whom are purebred and some of whom are not, (the dogs, not the friends.) They had generally advised us to get the same kind of dog they had, but none of them said much about the difference between purebred and other dogs. I have a cousin who raises golden retrievers, and I was surprised when she said labradoodles weren't a real breed. Some internet research opened my eyes to how the kind of prejudice that exists about people also exists about dogs. Here are typical quotes from Rui's ancestral organizations.

A Labradoodle is nothing more than an expensive mongrel.... These crossbreds are a deliberate attempt to mislead the public with the idea that there is an advantage to these designer dogs. The crossbred dogs are prone to all of the genetic disease of both breeds and offer none of the advantages that owning a purebred dog has to offer.
Labrador Retriever Club of America

Do not ever allow your stud dog to be bred to a bitch of another breed. If you are a member of a breed club, this could put you in line for charges being brought against you. Why? This is not responsible

Poodle Club of America

It sounded like General Jack D. Ripper bemoaning the dilution of the purity of the white race in "Dr. Strangelove".

But there is of course one major difference between humans and dogs in regards to racial prejudice: dogs are too smart to believe this nonsense. When I take Rui out for a walk, he meets both pure-bred and crossbred dogs, and despite what Ms. Molly claimed, there's no difference in how they treat one another based on breed. Pure breeds aren't snotty, or hostile to "lesser breeds without the law". Rui is attracted to poodles and other doodles. When I took him to his first "doodle romp" I was amused how all forty doodles shared a particular way of playing (more batting of paws than most dogs). It's very clear that such purebred prejudice is a human foible, not a canine one. Dogs intuitively know what Wikipedia says, "As all dog breeds have been derived from mixed-breed dog populations, the term 'purebred' has meaning only with respect to a certain number of generations". Dog breeds in their current sense only go back to 1873, and the English Kennel Club. And current DNA research has proven the concept of races among humans is just as invalid as it is among dogs.

When I taught high school, I often noticed how attractive the students from mixed racial backgrounds were. In a number of Native American spiritual traditions, including the one I practice, the term "rainbow peoples" is used for those whose ancestors are different colours. It's a term of respect, and if one has to have names for races, it's as good as any. But it seems clear to continue pretending these hugely artificial constructs have a real objective meaning is both biologically wrong and sociologically harmful. Darwin (who didn't believe in races) pointed out that there were two, three, four, five, eleven, sixteen, twenty-two, or sixty-three races according to the current experts of his time.

If, as Raymund Nash said, "Horse sense is what keeps horses from betting on what people will do," then maybe "dog sense" is what keeps dogs from caring about races and pedigree. Surely it's finally time for humans to put those divisions behind us, even at the cost of being shunned by the Poodle Society of America, or their racist equivalents.

Brave words, but all prejudices are easier to disown than to remove. I noticed a few weeks later how when someone (often male) asked (in a certain tone), "What kind of dog is that?" I'd casually answer that Rui was 5/8 poodle, and 3/8 lab. Now this is true (his maternal grandmother – a first generation labradoodle – was crossed with a full poodle, so his mother was 3/4 poodle, while his father was a labradoodle), though pedantic. But the underlying message was Rui was not a mutt, that his breeding was as deliberate as any purebred dog. Given my earlier comments on racism, I have to acknowledge there's a whiff of hypocrisy in the air here. All I ask is you don't hold it against Rui.

Racism isn't the only prejudice humans project onto dogs. I was walking Rui in our back alley, and encountered a neighbour walking his dog. He was a man in his fifties, whom I mentally called Popeye, as his weatherbeaten face reminded me of the childhood cartoon I once watched. We hadn't talked much, but as we both had dogs we started chatting while our dogs did the canine equivalent. Suddenly Popeye grabbed his dog and jerked him away from Rui. I asked what was wrong.

"They were kissing each other," he said, "and they're both boy dogs!"

I looked at Rui, then back at Popeye, and decided this was a battle I wasn't going to take on. It would take more than spinach to cure Popeye of this particular disease. I suddenly came to a deeper appreciation of the old joke, "The more I see of people, the more I like my dog." Rui and I just turned and walked off down the alley in the opposite direction.

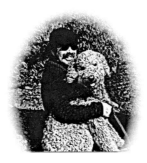

9. A Christmas Meditation

"What must I do, to tame you?" asked the little prince.
"You must be very patient," replied the fox. "First you will
sit down at a little distance from me--like that--in the grass.
I shall look at you out of the corner of my eye, and you will
say nothing. Words are the source of misunderstandings.
But you will sit a little closer to me, every day . . ."

Antoine de Saint-Exupéry *The Little Prince*

S ometimes distance did give perspective. That was what I was thinking early Christmas morning, 2006, as I sat by myself at the ancient dining room table in Carversville, Pennsylvania, where Diana and I had come to share Christmas with Brenda, her 88 year old mother. Brenda had always been a dog person, but her strong sense of how things in her house ought to be seemed as though it would conflict a bit too dramatically with our four month old puppy's innate affinity towards chaos. Diana had prepared me extensively before I was ready to meet Brenda, and we agreed that Rui's preparation was not yet comparable. So he had been left to languish at a kennel in Toronto, while I thought the tranquil early morning (before the others awoke, before the gifts were opened, but after the coffee was made) would be a fine time to look back on the first two months of my dogged experience and explore both the reflections from its surface, and what I could see of the depths beneath.

I had started reading much more extensively about dogs of course, beginning with puppy guides. My favourite was "The Art of Raising a Puppy", by the Monks of New Skete, particularly as Rui chewed its paper cover off, and left the hardcover tattooed with toothmarks. That gave it an air of deeper authenticity. It had a gentleness and humanity that made me warm to it, as did their other book, "How to Be Your Dog's Best Friend". I reread Harlan Ellison's "Ahbhu", a short piece about the death of his dog, the one who inspired his brilliant novelette "A Boy and His Dog". I'd also read "Marley and Me", an entertainingly sentimental NY Times best seller about an almost untrainable Labrador; "White Dog", Romain Gary's heartrendingly cynical commentary on America, racism, and the futility of hope; "My Dog Tulip", an indulgently loving paean to a British alsatian; and reread Jack London's "The Call of the Wild". For me the most genuinely insightful and moving of them all was Mark Doty's "Dog Years", his exploration of the meaning of the last years in the lives and deaths of his dogs.

My relationship with my neighbourhood had changed. Our house was a few doors south of Bloor Street, the main east-west artery in downtown Toronto. I often walked along that street, to buy groceries or go to convenient local restaurants, or to get on the subway on the other side of Bloor. But the rest of the residential neighbourhood was something I passed through on my way to somewhere more interesting. Now I knew about the back alleys that lay between the main streets, and the motley assortment of garages that opened onto them. I had discovered local parks, and where the holes were in fences that opened onto the railroad tracks, and the fine walking trails next to them. From the very first Rui was surprisingly indifferent to the occasional freight trains that rumbled by. My local area had become a place I experienced, rather than just a piece of geography around our house.

Rui had changed my relationship with other people too. As I walked him I identified other people walking their dogs as Members of our Tribe (MOT) and we approached and made friendly conversation about names, ages and breeds while our dogs did the equivalent, only with more sniffing. (Though afterwards, I confess, I only remembered them as Sophie's mother, or Akita's father.) I learned – what I wish I had known in my twenties – that a cute puppy was a most powerful catalyst for starting conversations with women. And I was amazed to learn how many people were terrified of dogs, hurriedly crossing a street to avoid any chance of canine proximity. While I had known some of my friends had dogs, that was a trivial irrelevance on the order of knowing which of them had foreign cars as opposed to domestic. Now some ancient and almost desiccated friendships suddenly blossomed again, and friends in the country who were always a bit too far away to visit seemed to have Eden-like vistas, hugely appealing. And of course there was Suzanne, our dog-trainer, who had become my guru in canine matters, all-knowing and wise and available for consultation whenever Rui and I reached an impasse over which of us was Alpha and which was Beta.

Relationships with some other people had become more distant, those who disliked dogs or feared their allergies might have been triggered by non-allergenic Rui. When I talked to some friends about how owning a dog had changed my life, or tried to share the new discovery or challenge that particular day had brought, I saw some people glaze over and wait eagerly for a chance to divert the conversation to more important and deeper things, such as the real books they'd read, or recent political developments in the Afghan hinterland. Suddenly I understood at a deeper and more visceral level the frustration of women who stayed at home to raise children, and their feelings when ex-friends talked of "real jobs" or of what was happening in the world. It felt as though those people were valuing passively viewing the giant plasma screen on which the world's events were displayed as somehow outranking the creative shaping of new life.

As well, my relationship with others had been modified by the imposition of an unprecedented and near-absolute discipline. Rui must be fed, must be walked, must be allowed outside at regular intervals to do his business. Diana had (as she had always known she would) fallen in love with Rui as much as I had, and fully shared the tasks. But spontaneous decisions to go see a movie, or to leave the house with no idea when we'd be back weren't possible any more. Nor was it an option to return home late from an evening out and fall into bed; Rui had to be fed, then taken out a half hour later. I was like a needle on a shaken compass, swinging around to all directions, but always feeling a slightly greater pull to north. In the midst of the new Spiderman film with my nephew Sam, or while discussing with friends whether we should or should not join the protest next Sunday, I suddenly felt Rui at home in the kitchen, alone, wanting food and company and wondering when his Alpha Male would return and free him from his leaden tedium. In the past an evening's social pleasure was to be savoured and drained to its last drops, like an 18 year old McCallum; now it got left sooner rather than later, like skipping the tedious naming of the members of the band on a concert recording.

And when I came home, at the front door I would see Rui's shadow falling from where he lay pressed against the door. I opened it and he was always pleased to see me, licking my hand, eagerly accepting the belly-rubs I offered him, enthusiastic as always about almost anything I did if it involved him. (Grooming was still something to be endured rather than cherished; I empathized with how he felt about that.) He was always a quiet dog, barking only when he wanted attention, or in excitement when it became clear I was going out and might take him if I were reminded. But neither visitors, nor strange sounds provoked barks, and his only growls came playfully when we were tugging on opposite ends of a pull-toy.

In the seven weeks we'd shared he had started to develop a super-ego, though he was still predominantly a creature ruled by his id, his animal nature. But that super-ego, the sense of what he ought to do, was slowly starting to show. A week before the Carversville trip Rui was running loose in our backyard, and I went out to call him. He immediately stopped running, crouched down facing me about ten yards away, and barked fiercely. It was clear that he both knew I wanted him to come to me, and he didn't want to, for fear I would take him into the boring house and abandon him in the kitchen, the only room over which he had free reign at that point. I called him again, and he pulled himself a yard closer and repeated the bark. After each subsequent call he would slowly drag himself along the ground a bit closer till after about five minutes he touched my hands with his muzzle, then leapt quickly away. I stayed motionless and called him, until finally he surrendered to duty, and came up to me, letting himself be petted and rubbed as a reward. That pull between his wanting to run away, and his clear sense that he ought to come when called was fascinating to watch play out.

Our main bone of contention came over the concept of heeling, which was ultimately a question of whose interests were going to determine the walk: my boring and tedious desire to plod in a straight line down the sidewalk, or his excited curiosity at exploring the rich world of a thousand overlaid smells pulling him off in all directions. Secondary differences were about other people, whom he invariably wanted to get to know (more so if they were children) and other dogs whom he found almost as exciting. Owners of these dogs were less disturbed than the parents of babies in strollers when Rui tried to leap up and lick them. He was not yet, alas, a Good Canine Citizen. He was always indifferent in puppydom to cats, birds, and squirrels, any of which might have provoked a mild curiosity, but not any great desire to pursue when they fled. He walked past a cat at this time not even noticing as it puffed itself up, raised its tail and prepared for a fight; he was indifferent as it preened in victory when he had gone past. And often, I would see other dogs coming long before he noticed them, caught up as he was with a fascinating smell that kept his nose down.

Of course he did have a far superior sense of smell to mere humans'. He would nose at a pocket in which there was hidden a dog treat, even though it was still wrapped in sealed plastic. He distinguished instantly between hamburger coming out of the freezer for him, and the lowly veggie-burgers Diana or I preferred. And he went into an anticipatory frenzy while that meat was being defrosted and cooked. Perhaps it was lucky we were vegetarian as Rui never had to face the disappointment of smelling meat which wouldn't find its way to his bowl.

Walking with him was what it must be like to be colour blind and walk through a museum with a friend who's not. You're both in front of the same things, but you're sadly aware that she's seeing a whole part of the world you can't. I was walking Rui down St. Clarens Street, a block from home, and we passed an old blue couch someone was throwing out. It was well-worn and faded, and I glanced at it and would have walked on, but Rui was very interested, and methodically sniffed all the cushions, and the crevices between them, and the back of the couch before he was ready to walk on. He didn't seem as though he was tracking down food bits, or learning about another dog (he probably would have peed on the couch if it had another dog's scent.) But when in a few minutes he was ready to leave it, I marveled at how he now had acquired a whole history of the couch and its ex-occupants that wasn't accessible to me.

At times that world of scent completely overwhelmed Rui. He walked into a telephone pole once while his nose was to the ground intently following a fascinating smell. In an open field, he'd look like a textbook diagram of Brownian motion as he went back and forth and around following the exact path, I suspect, that something else did a few hours earlier. I'd become curious that dogs didn't catch colds; perhaps it was because while losing one's sense of smell for a few days is merely an inconvenience to a human, it could be a fatal handicap to a wolf. But Rui never had a runny or plugged nose, and rarely sneezed.

He existed in a world of body and emotion, and to learn to communicate with him, to teach him to behave as we want him to, was a fascinating challenge. All the more so because of how much I'd always taught through intellect, and it was of course utterly useless to say to Rui that if he heeled as I wanted him to while we walked to the park, then he'd get to run free there. The challenge was greater because training had to be done without diminishing Rui's spirit, his friendly joy in all that was around him. But slowly we had learned to communicate with each other. When he was frightened by a big dog barking fiercely as we walked past a garage he'd come close to me, clearly aware I was his protector. So I started to learn to communicate in his language, both understanding more of what he wanted me to know and finding ways to let him know what I wanted him to do.

Of course Rui wasn't human, and training a puppy wasn't like having a baby, for all the similarities that having a dependent living creature come into one's life might have held. But when Diana and I went home after taking him to the kennel, the house seemed empty, and even the joy of staying late in bed, or leaving the papers by the edge of the table and not having to close the kitchen door behind us seemed small exchange for having such a diminished pack.

As I sat at the Christmas table writing, I suddenly remembered the passage in Antoine de Saint Exupéry, when the fox persuaded the little prince to tame him. The fox said, "…if you tame me, it will be as if the sun came to shine on my life. I shall know the sound of a step that will be different from all the others. Other steps send me hurrying back underneath the ground. Yours will call me, like music, out of my burrow. And then look: you see the grain-fields down yonder? I do not eat bread. Wheat is of no use to me. The wheat fields have nothing to say to me. And that is sad. But you have hair that is the color of gold. Think how wonderful that will be when you have tamed me! The grain, which is also golden, will bring me back the thought of you."

Before Rui I would have seen dogs on the street and nothing more. Now I looked at them, and they reminded me of him, and I felt happy because I had a dog who loved me. In three days we would be back at the kennel, our pack would be complete again, and we would go on learning more about and from each other and how we shared our lives. And I suspected, accurately, for all the joys that a fine Christmas trip to Brenda had brought us, the moment of reuniting would be the greatest pleasure of all.

*

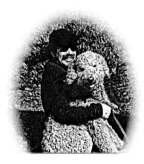

10. In Sickness and in Health

"It is by disease that health is pleasant."

Heraclitus

After we returned from our week in the States, Diana and I ransomed Rui from Birchmount Kennels from whose marketing department he'd earned an A+ on his amusingly formal report card. The next six days seemed like a microcosm of the ups and downs of life with a dog. Rui seemed happy to be home, but he was happy in general so that wasn't noteworthy. We celebrated the reuniting of our pack with a long and enjoyable walk through High Park, taking advantage of the uncovered grass in an unseasonably warm January. Rui revealed a habit he would always have by suddenly dipping his head while walking across grass and doing a forward somersault. Then he lay on his back with all four limbs waving skyward and ecstatically wriggled and squirmed, in what our nephew Sam called, "a grass seizure". It seemed a very Zen behaviour: full of joy at life and utterly in the present.

The next day he was happy to go for a long walk with our extended pack: Amy and Mo, (Sam's mothers) and Sam through the long dog-friendly ravine of Cedarvale park Sam was in charge of his leash. This was the first time he had felt comfortable in control of Rui, and both of them seemed happy with the process, even if Rui would have preferred to explore the mud wallow more fully than Sam allowed. The adults unanimously supported Sam.

But on the drive home, Rui vomited, just over the edge of his car carpet and did so again in the yard at home. He also started coughing and sneezing and didn't jump up as usual when I came into the kitchen. Instead he lay on his side and weakly licked once at my hand instead of softly and energetically biting it, which is his usual greeting. At this first intimation of canine mortality, January suddenly got colder, and less welcoming. On the verge of panicking, I went and got his favourite freeze-dried liver treat and held it out from across the room. Rui jumped to his feet, bounded over, and snatched it from my hand. Liver treats are clearly a useful medical indicator, and when he collapsed again after devouring this one, I was distinctly less worried about his imminent death. But he still was as sick as a dog.

Rui came with Paddy's two year warranty against any genetic disease, such as hip dysplasia, that he might develop. But dogs, like people, get more sickly as they age, and friends had told of having to make horrible decisions over whether to pay for expensive treatments for their aging pets, or have them put down. Canada's medical system avoids having to make such decisions about people, and I didn't want to ever have to make them over Rui. Therefore he was insured: for about $40 a month he's covered for up to $30,000 for sickness or injury, over the course of his life. So between his early shots and this insurance, Rui was armed against the slings and arrows of outrageous fortune as much as he could be. We'd had him vaccinated against kennel cough before he went to the kennel, an expense not covered by the insurance as it was preventative.

But despite the vaccination, kennel cough still seemed the logical candidate for his sickness. Internet research explained it usually goes away, but without treatment terrible things sometimes happened. So it was back to the vet, where I learned Rui had a slight fever and that the normal temperature for dogs is 2° C (or 3.6° F) higher than humans, which explained why he always felt warm. I managed to use the first $100 of Rui's $30,000 on a two week course of antibiotics. I declined the purchase of beef-flavoured doughnuts to hide the pills in (I knew they wouldn't be covered) and instead used tiny slits in mandarin orange segments (which Rui loved).

The antibiotics worked; two days later he was recovered enough that we had a forty–five minute walk in the morning, and invented a new game in the fenced park a half mile from home in the afternoon. It consisted of my trying to catch Rui while he ran in circles around me. Three weeks earlier I had been able to outrun him, it was impressive how impossible that was now. His energy was clearly back. On the way home he suddenly darted past me holding a bra in his mouth, which seemed a pretty slick move for a guy lacking opposable thumbs. Happily for my neighbourhood relationships, a backwards glance showed no outraged woman in hot pursuit. It was just detritus in the alley, with the story of how it came to be abandoned buried forever in the unknown.

Rui and I most bonded during our afternoon walks. He was starting to become more responsive, and I was learning more deeply who he was and how to communicate with him. That afternoon our walk was amazing—Rui showed five new behaviours. When I went to the back yard to put the leash on he played "Shy", which had become one of his favourite backyard games. The rules of Shy seemed to be that Rui had to come very close to me and then leap away when I tried to touch him. He appeared to get extra points if he could touch my hand with his nose and still not get caught.

He has always had a persistent fondness for pushing any rule's edge. When given a boundary, he'd stay where he'd been told to, but surreptitiously slide his nose, or a paw just across the boundary line. Then he'd look, innocently, at us. It was a behaviour I had seen a lot in high school students, who also liked pushing the boundaries. And as with them, I probably let it slide more with Rui than

I should have. But this day when he played Shy, I said "Rui, come here," sternly and he immediately came and stood still to let me put the leash on. When we walked, he heeled or stayed with a slack leash 85% of the hour, neither pulling nor tugging. And when I stopped, he'd sit at my feet. I started standing still when a person or group walked towards us, and Rui would sit down and let them go by. It was a new and delightful behaviour.

On this walk, he only did what I most hated once, which was to start biting at the leash and leaping at my hands, snapping and growling. He did wag his tail, so it appeared to be somewhere between a game and a tantrum, but I felt it was wrong and would become furious. I had developed two ways of stopping it. One was to have a major distraction such as a squeaky toy at hand, which always worked, but was not always possible. The other sure way was to do the "Alpha Roll": I grabbed Rui, rolled him onto his back and glared into his eyes. This always worked, but seemed extreme, particularly to passing children who wondered why this bad man was beating up the cute puppy and to whom they should report it. The Monks had advised me that the Alpha roll was appropriate for discipline, (though in later editions they would change their mind). But that afternoon when he leapt at the leash, I just said "Rui, No!" and he stopped and went back to heeling docilely.

Then when we came back home, Rui sat on the front porch lying across my lap, alertly watching people walk. He didn't bite at my fingers once, and enjoyed being petted and praised. He sat there quite calmly for a half hour, through the fading of our new warm January sunset. All those new behaviours in a single walk! While I was being changed by living with Rui, his changes were out pacing mine by as much as he could now outrun me. I felt very pleased, as though my ability to train him was suddenly reality–based rather than faith–based. I felt maybe all the books and instructions were going to work after all.

It seemed strange all these behaviours appeared on the same day (the heeling had been coming, but the others were all new). Perhaps he'd known for a while what we wanted him to do, and just decided on that day to start. Maybe he had been afraid we'd leave him in the kennel forever if he didn't behave, or perhaps they had better trainers in the kennel who knew how to train him? Or could it be that the antibiotics had some amazing behavioural side effects? Though if that were the case, Big Pharma could sell them wholesale to pet owners, who'd buy anything, (as my purchase of dog insurance showed). But forty–eight hours earlier, as I had watched him cough heavily on the kitchen floor, I wouldn't have believed we'd be in this place so soon. Like Rui, beside me on the porch, I was one happy puppy.

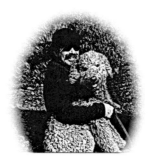

II. iPod and iDog

"Hey, mister deejay, won't cha hear my last prayer?
Hey, ho, rock 'n roll, deliver me from nowhere."

Bruce Springsteen, *Open All Night*

No longer teaching high school had some surprising side effects. One was that I lost the hour of foreground listening to music that had been the sound track to my daily commute. As a child of the sixties, I had always believed the right music might transform my life again. (I was at the first Beatles concert in Canada, saw The Who perform *Tommy* from the front row in Boston, was at Hendrix's last concert on the Isle of Wight, and blissed out to more Grateful Dead concerts than I could remember, for a number of reasons.) Generally, Diana didn't share my taste for loud high-energy music, so the car had been a space where I could indulge without bothering her. And now that hour of music was gone.

I found technology offered an answer, as technology so often has in my life. Shortly after I left teaching high school, I got an iPod. After it was fully loaded, it could play music for 32 days before it started to repeat. It was a wonderful new toy that played any music or radio podcasts I wanted. I could plug it into a Bose sound dock and have a high end portable music player that was smaller than my Panasonic boom-box of ten years ago, but had almost as good sound as my best speakers. The iPod's main use was to provide a soundtrack for long walks around Toronto, helping me get some exercise while allowing me to lose myself in music.

So these walks became my new way of foregrounding music. I loved being able to listen in a way I rarely did at home, where music was most often a background soundtrack. I loved how dead easy it was to move the slider on my headphones to quiet the music when it was time to ask the barrista for a grande half-sweet vanilla latte. I'd blissfully drift along in my world, floating in sound, navigating the real world on autopilot.

While walking, I might suddenly reach a deeper understanding of a Tom Waits' lyric, or develop a grand obsession with Algerian Rai music. When I was skiing with my iPod, I would dance down the hill, turning in time to the rhythm of the playlist I'd selected for that day. And when I'd get tired and footsore, a livelier selection would help me keep going. But listening to the iPod was largely a way to get exercise without having to be involved with the exercise itself, without having to be involved with my body. I might write up my new discoveries online, or share them with friends, but my peer group wasn't as passionate as it was in the 60's about music, when it seemed as though each album were a potentially life-transforming gift from the music gods to be savoured slowly and debated furiously amongst the rockerati. So while my pleasure in musical involvement was still being fed, it was an isolated one.

But all that suddenly and completely ended when most of my walking became with Rui. In the iPod wandering days, the white ibuds blaring in my ears carried me away so completely sometimes I'd walk fifteen minutes without noticing a single thing about the part of the city through which I'd gone. Setting out from home meant having no idea where I would wind up. I'd walk into strange neighbourhoods, go for a few hours into a new part of Toronto, and then hop on the TTC to come home feeling tired. With Rui, walking around the neighbourhood along an increasingly familiar set of back alleys, over and over, was my new routine. It was winter, so we tried to avoid the streets, not because of people and cars, but because of the winter salt that melted ice but irritated a dog's feet. All walks had to be there and back again, as Rui was far too attracted to people, and too eager to get to know them, for buses to yet be an option.

But changes in route were just the wrapping. The core of the difference was under that, in the activity itself.

I couldn't listen to an iPod when walking him. I needed my sense of hearing, and wearing headphones blocked out the world. Indeed, walking with Rui at the end of a leash instead of an iPod at the end of my headphones was hardly the same activity. The leash needed to be constantly watched and untangled, which was more challenging because I liked having him on the six metre variety. I needed to be fully present and alert not only to what he was doing in any moment, but to what he might do in the next. It was a constant test pitting my superior sense of sight against his superior sense of smell. A child coming towards us, an abandoned Tim Horton's cup on the sidewalk, dog excrement: leading him out of temptation was all part of my Godlike duties in his life.

There was a walk he wanted to take, which was meandering, and involved with smells, and had lots of noshing en route. There was the walk I wanted to take, which was straight, proceeded at a constant pace, and didn't have any eating from the ground included. I could have Rui take my walk, mostly, only by being involved with him. Short quick tugs on his leash alerted him to change what he was doing. If I didn't give those little tugs, he'd strain and pull and I had to yank him, leading him to attack the leash. While he still would heel some of the time, that earlier January walk on which he'd heeled now seemed more of a coming attraction than a permanent change.

Walking Rui was a mercurial activity. One day, as we walked sedately to Dufferin Grove Park, he spotted a group of pigeons for whom some kind soul had left stale bread rolls. Suddenly he was obsessed and fascinated and only the fact I outweighed him let me get him past those rolls. Two days earlier I'd been talking to Sam as we walked Rui. I wasn't paying attention, and suddenly I had to force Rui's jaws open to get him to release a particularly delectable slimy bun. He fought to keep it, but was good-natured when I won: no snarls or bites.

And that was the heart of the difference, having to be fully present and responsive and involved with him. Sometimes I'd let him play and meander, while sometimes it was a training walk; I needed to be sensitive to both his moods and mine as I communicated to him which kind of walk we were on. When we walked past a garage, and a dog started barking inside, Rui would quite reasonably want to stop and listen. He gradually came to accept my desire he not wander out onto city streets. Walking with him, I realized, was part of our on-going dialogue, one that would shape the adult dog he'd become and the behaviour I'd live with for years as a result of what I did on these early walks. This was a new way for what I did to matter and be meaningful, which was one of the pieces I most missed after leaving teaching.

When I had started teaching, my subjects were Physics and Maths. By the time I ended, they were English and World Religions. Changing fields was a way to get more involvement with the students, and to learn along with them. The fifth time through quadratic equations, I wasn't learning a lot from my students, or much new about myself. World Religions is infinite in scope, and each student brought a unique perspective and experience to the course. Our interaction deepened the experience of the course, for me and for them, because their views mattered.

It was curious how the change from iPod to iDog paralleled that change of teaching subjects. The iPod was like a certain kind of math/science teacher, the one who focused on the subject and ignored the students. It played exactly the same way whether I was listening and intent, or off woolgathering. Rui and I interacted as we walked, and that made me focus and be present with him. I had to not just be in my head, but in my body, and always dealing with my emotional reactions to behaviour that wasn't what I wanted. There were no assignments given for the next day, and no discussions about what happened the day before. Walking with Rui was a different kind of gift, one through which he taught me to be more present and aware as fully as I was teaching him. Teachers come, I was starting to learn, in a variety of forms.

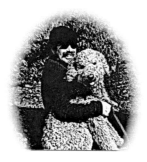

12. The Law of the Leash

"A leash is only a rope with a noose at both ends."

Ayn Rand, *The Fountainhead*

Rui had been with us for three and a half months. We'd spent time apart during Christmas, but aside from that we had walked him twice a day, every day. Diana was doing about two walks a week, so I had done the other twelve, which worked out to about 165 walks. Usually Rui walked on a short two metre leash, though sometimes in a park, he got a six metre training leash. But (except for enclosed and fenced areas) never had Rui or I walked together without one.

Some dog owners were puzzled I didn't let him off leash in parks, but I feared Rui would happily bolt, and whether the other dogs or the plastic bag floating on the wind were on the other side of the street or not would make no difference. And his penchant for greeting small children by leaping on them and licking their faces wasn't always welcomed by either the children or their parents, however much joy it might have brought to their parents' lawyers. In a fenced area, Rui would only come half the time when he was called. So all

I could see at this point was our walking together bound by the law of the leash, me with my wrist in one of the nooses and Rui with his head in the other. The dream of walking freely with an unleashed dog at my side seemed very far away and unreal.

And of course my head was in the noose too. Every morning between 7 and 8, every afternoon between 3 and 5, I would get down a leash, put on some boots and a jacket, tell Rui to stop barking (he got excited at the possibility of going outside) and head out. I found it mildly terrifying to contemplate doing this every day, more or less, for the next fifteen years, totalling around 10,000 walks. Living in the city with a dog was a far more absolute discipline than anything I had ever had in my life before: teaching was a mere 200 days out of the 365. And one could take sick days, if needed. I had imagined leaving teaching in high school would set me free; instead I was feeling the constriction of the far less flexible regimen I had created for myself.

But not walking Rui certainly wasn't a viable option; one day I had come downstairs at three, and thought, "He doesn't need two walks every day, I'm exhausted, I won't go today", and headed back upstairs to the computer. A loud crashing sound a half hour later brought me back down. I realized that before he had pulled down all the beer bottles and chewed up their cases, he had pulled open the drawer with the 100 tea candles I'd bought from IKEA, and chewed up most of those. And a bag of patterned paper napkins I hadn't thrown out because they were a gift could now be thrown out, after they'd been swept up, and before we went for the walk. Instant karma had indeed gotten me, and pretty damn quickly too.

At this stage one could have held a fine debate over who was actually in charge on these walks. While Rui would heel on some days, on others he would tug frantically when he wanted to go faster, or investigate some particularly odoriferous tidbit that lay buried beneath the snow's crust, just out of reach. I would make the major decisions about which park we'd walk to, or when it was time to head home. He would get to snap at me when he didn't approve of the decision to go home. I'd get to do a "down", in which I stood on his leash so he had to lie unmoving for a few minutes after he had snapped at me, at which point he gnawed at my ankle. Those were the cascading inevitabilities of our daily walks. Perhaps the answer to who was in charge was pretty clearly Rui, considering he got to poop anywhere he wanted, while I got to scurry around with a little plastic bag picking up his offerings.

I knew he was controlled with the longer leash, but pretended the longer leash gave him freedom. It was the same as when I was teaching. Then, I pretended to have the freedom to do what I wanted in my classroom by breaking a few school rules like letting kids eat in class, or play computer games. But really I was controlled by the school, who would have intervened with absolute power had some serious tenet been transgressed. But I was probably even less likely to do that than Rui was to break his rules, which he did instantly if a piece of pizza appeared from under a melting snowbank. Strangely, indoors at home, he'd let me take anything away from him: food, bones, toys. But outside the controls were off. It was a dog–eat–dough world out there.

My students probably thought my classroom was pretty lenient, but of course we all had our respective leashes so thoroughly attached there was no chance of breaking the rules.. The most effective leashes are always the ones you don't even notice you're wearing. I'd internalized the school board's rules so well I believed I was free to do what I wanted, so well they could trust me to make the right decisions.

And leashes did give you a certain feeling of security. You knew where you were with a leash, whether you were walking a dog, doing your daily job, or swinging from a gibbet at the end of one. The future might be unknown, but a leash always let you know exactly where you were relative to at least one other point. Was that why after I left teaching I had found ways to be in the world with my writing course (and the weekly responses to my students' writing that it required) or with my newsletter (and the weekly amassing

61

of stories, layout, and publishing that it required)? Teaching is a hugely prescribed occupation. In September, had I been asked what I would be doing at 10:30 May 14th I could have figured out which class I would be teaching at that hour, and roughly where I'd be in that course at the time. So perhaps it wasn't surprising that after over thirty years a leash was comfortable to me.

Rui was certainly less comfortable. But I did know consistency was the key, just as in a classroom. When I had become more skilled at teaching, the need for overt discipline lessened. My students knew what I wanted, and where the boundaries were, so their leashes didn't need constant tugging. This process had started with Rui, and it lessened my fears for the future. We both had started to learn what the other wanted. He was leaping up less on passersby because I really disliked it and yanked his leash when he did that; I walked next to any deep snow we passed, and let him leap into it and stick his head in to explore what lay beneath the surface because that so clearly delighted him. And there were times when we walked in harmony, neither of us pulling the other, both of us enjoying it. He'd watch when I went on one side or the other of a lamp post, and follow me; I'd watch when he found a particularly interesting set of messages dribbled at the base of a tree, and let him absorb them in detail.

Rui had recently acquired the doggy habit of stopping at telephone poles and fire hydrants, and sniffing for a long while to absorb the information there. It seemed for dogs pee-mail served the same function email does for us; there are some updates from friends, some important news, and a lot of boring spam you weren't interested in. Sometimes Rui would add his two scents worth, and when he wouldn't, he'd sniff meticulously up and down for a minute, and then turn to me, ready to go on. Those were the moments we transcended the law of the leash, when we were just two creatures out together exploring the world, when the good noose became like no noose at all.

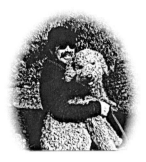

13. Parks and Socialization

"We don't need no education
We don't need no thought control
...Hey, teacher, leave us kids alone."

Pink Floyd, *Another Brick in the Wall, Part II*

One of the lessons city dogs need to learn is to get along with other dogs whom they pass on the street, or encounter in the adjacent back yard. This socialization happens in dog parks. And, as Rui grew bigger, the days when I could run fast enough to exhaust him had clearly passed. He needed more exercise, and so it was time for him to learn how to cope with the world of dogs, and people other than Diana and me. When at three months he got the shots which allowed him to safely play with dogs, we entered into the process of finding the right dog park.

The process was similar to choosing a school for a child. Like a pair of protective parents, we were concerned he not fall in with the wrong crowd, a group of rough dogs who would bully him, or whom he'd join with to bully other dogs. Like students' parents on a school planning council, dog owners naturally become a political interest group, meeting at park planning sessions, and wanting more space and time for their dogs just as the parents want more computers for their children.

Similarly to how parents may find their social life increasingly filled by parents of their children's schoolmates, choosing a dog park is also selecting a social group. As people tended to walk their dogs at the same time every day, social issues became part of our choice, along with the more obvious questions of proximity, size, and the number, age, and kind of other dogs who were usually there at that time of the day. Mercifully, at least there was less paperwork if we decided to change from one park to another.

Toronto is a green enough city to have made this a pleasingly complex choice. The rivers that once flowed south into Lake Ontario are now largely dammed or underground, leaving a web of lovely narrow ravine parks all over the city. A map of Toronto looks as though a child had dipped their fingers in green paint and carelessly drawn their hand from north of the city down to the lake, dripping spots here and there next to their spidery lines. The jewel of the city's parks was High Park, over one and a half square kilometres of gloriously varied terrain, and the only park I had regularly visited in my pre-dog days, when I happily played one of its frisbee golf courses. It also had the largest off leash area of any park, which seemed attractive till our first visit when I realized that meant big dogs and their owners tended to come there, and Rui was as intimidated as a six year old being taken into a high school. He wasn't ready for either big dogs or off leash areas yet.

So his first walks were to an enclosed park about a kilometre away. Diana and I christened it the chocolate factory, because across the tracks on its western side was a large Cadbury's plant, so if the wind were westerly you could gain a pound or two just by inhaling. I liked it there, partially because it was enclosed by a fence so I could let go of the leash and let Rui run without fearing he wouldn't return. And there I first regularly met other dog people: Sophia, seventyish, and Princess, a slow moving beagle who would tolerate Rui jumping all over her, then give a serious bark that backed him off; or Steven, an art teacher with whom Rui loved to play, even if his two dogs were utterly indifferent to mine. I liked Steven but the dog chemistry simply wasn't there.

I explored two other local parks, Dufferin Grove and Dovercourt Park. But neither of them had official dog areas so if animal control officers were ever to come by, we would all be fined $255 if our dogs were running free, or on a leash over two metres in length. Fortunately this never happened; unfortunately it was perhaps because there often weren't any dogs exercising at seven in the morning or three thirty in the afternoon, the times I usually took Rui out. So I cast our net further afield after a few months, looking for a larger school to provide better canine education for our youngster.

Then I found Bickford Park, to which I usually drove rather that spending an hour walking there along busy Bloor Street. Garrison Creek once flowed through it, but what's left now is a large bowl, with high sides, where dogs can run around in the centre legally. There were almost always dogs there, and Rui was happy to play with any of them, even Max, an aggressive unneutered beagle who was shunned by most of the other dogs and their owners. (It's the same $255 fine to have an unneutered male past six months of age off leash in Toronto; too much testosterone ends up producing too many dog fights.)

It amazed me how much Rui's play varied with the kind of dog. With other poodle-related breeds, he slapped at their heads or bodies with his paws, and they responded in kind. Then they chased each other around. With more solid dogs, like Chompsky, a golden retriever, or Domi, a young bulldog, Rui would wrestle trying to pin the other dog, or to get out from under the pin he'd been subject to. Ten minutes of serious dog play gave Rui more exercise than a half hour of walking with me.

And I got to chat to dog owners while our dogs played. It was my first time regularly meeting with a community of other owners, and as we all had at least one interest in common, the conversations started easily, whether it was talking politics with Chompsky's people, or hockey with Domi's.

Sorauren, about the same distance away, was another favourite dog park. The canine part was a large open space next to a baseball diamond, and there were about half a dozen dogs of Rui's age whom I'd often find there. Over the next months, they all became close friends and leapt on each other with barks of joy when they'd meet. And there too were equally friendly owners with whom to chat as we shared the spring warmth. But the problem with both Bickford and Sorauren was that I wasn't getting any exercise: while Rui romped, rolled, and raced with Keno (a high energy German Shepherd) I'd stand talking to Irene, Keno's owner. It was enjoyable to be part of a community and to get to know the different stories everyone had, but dog walks needed to involve some walking. That was one problem. The leash was another.

Almost all the other dogs were off leash, while Rui and I were still attached. So one day I took him to Sorauren, and decided to let him run and play untethered. First Heedra came by, a rottweiler on whom Rui had a crush. He licked her face over and over, which she tolerated. She was the only dog he ever did this with. Heedra played with him a bit, but she was six years old and not really into younger dogs and playing. All this time, he was near me, and would let me pet him as he rolled or strolled by.

Then Bullet, a chocolate lab, dropped his squeaky toy within Rui's lunge range, and that was it. Rui grabbed it, and was off. Bullet gave chase but eventually grew bored with that game, as Rui wasn't giving it back. So I tried to get him, but he was not going to allow that to happen. I called him, but he wouldn't come. He wouldn't even take his favorite treats when offered. When he wouldn't let me get close I ran away, and he ran after me – but stayed about ten feet away. Rui was faster and more agile than I was, and he knew I wanted to take his squeaky toy, and he knew that wasn't going to happen. And so it didn't.

Eventually it was time for Bullet's owner to leave, and he kindly and courteously said I could return the toy the next time we met. By now we'd been at the park about an hour and a half, and I was frustrated and at a loss for what to do. I thought of going to our Toyota Echo, and opening the hatchback for Rui to jump in, but going towards a busy street with a dog that was out of control seemed like upping the ante too much. I considered flying tackles, but as the ground was hard ice, at least one of us was going to get hurt. So I kept walking up to Rui, and telling him to sit, and he kept running away, and after a long while, he came too close to one of the other dog owners there who grabbed his collar, and that was that. He was a prisoner of the leash again. I led him to the car, and to home, and he surrendered the squeaky without protest (though with regret– he kept staring at the shelf where it awaited our next trip to Sorauren.)

Rui hadn't been fooled by my illusion of benign despotism. He understood control, and longed for its absence. He'd obey all my rules if I had power to enforce them, but only most of them if I didn't. While I wanted him to be obedient, part of me admired his independent spirit, and liked his consciousness that he didn't have to obey. I had admired high school students who dared to break the rules, and often got along better with them than some of my colleagues did. I was conflicted about Rui's independence, but I also knew his leash wouldn't be coming off again for a long time.

And finally I came back to High Park. Dog socialization, of course, happens in dog years, so rather than spending eight years in primary school, Rui was ready for high school in only eight months. By then he had reached his final weight of 25 kilograms, and could hold his own with bigger dogs. The larger park had more dogs and more owners, so there were more happy cases of an overlap between a dog Rui could play with and an owner Diana or I enjoyed talking to. And the kilometres of trails meant we could get exercise for ourselves as well as for our dog, sometimes walking alone with him in the more obscure corners of the park, sometimes walking with our gang through the dog off leash areas, where all of the dogs except Rui ran freely. Some day he too would, but only after he'd learned to come when called.

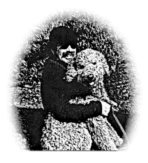

14. Entering Adolescence

"What have you done to the mirror?
What have you done to the floor?
Can't I go nowhere without you?
Can't I leave you alone any more?"

Randy Newman *Memo to my Son*

My innate attraction towards chaos has gotten me into trouble a few times. Most spectacularly, on a week long vision quest (a first nations' rite of passage ceremony) I cockily invited Eris, the Greek goddess of chaos, to come into my circle. She came, and after a year of major chaos in my life (end of marriage, major trouble at school, and a spate of unlikely injuries) I canoed out into the wilderness, built an altar, thanked Her for the teachings, and asked for a while to process them before getting any more. After that, things settled down. I suspected my attraction to trouble making students was another manifestation of that pull towards creative chaos. Rui was entering a phase in which he would test how deep my attraction still ran.

When I had anticipated living with a dog, and tried to imagine what that would be like, my visions had always been static. Walking the dog would be like this; training the dog would be like that. The dog and I would either have this kind of relationship or that kind, but always the images were fixed. And of course, the reality was nothing like that. Rui, at five months, was mercurial and moody and forced me even more to be in the present because of how little the past helped. Some of that was because he was growing and changing so fast, and some – I was coming to realize – might be just how puppies were.

When we weren't with him, Rui stayed alone in the kitchen, which we thought we'd fully dog-proofed. Everything edible or breakable had been moved off the lowest shelves, and child-proof latches had been put on the cupboards that contained potentially fatal cleansers. Then one day he broke the cinnamon shaker, a two dollar ceramic from our local Value Village. It was no great loss, except for the cinnamon all over the floor, and I had to go to the spice cupboard to get the requisite topping for my morning cappuccino. I didn't realize it at the time, but this was really foreshadowing. The shaker had been on the kitchen peninsula, a metre high; Rui had learned to stand up on his hind legs, and pull things off the counter.

I had thought, "Maybe the shaker had been too close to the edge," and moved everything to the centre before going upstairs to do some work. When I came down an hour later to take Rui out, he'd figured out how to pull out a lower drawer where we stored plastic bags, methodically shredded them, and left the remnants scattered over the floor. Usually he was lower energy after his walk, but, as I was later to discover, that day he had enough left to figure out how to reach the cubby where my wallet and keys used to be stored, to get the wallet down, extract all the money and credit cards, open the snap that keeps the subway tokens in, and scatter everything around the kitchen. He scorned the five and ten dollar bills, but did a dramatic job on a twenty, though I was later able to exchange it at a bank in its modified jigsaw puzzle and scotch tape form.

That day I had a luncheon date with an ex–colleague in Mississauga, and thought I had Rui-proofed the kitchen before leaving. Our Thai meal was fine (for a chain restaurant in a suburban mall) and it was a treat to see my friend again and hear stories of how she was riding this year's teaching cycle, even if it didn't seem hugely different from last year's model. There aren't many new student behaviours from year to year. By contrast, on returning I found Rui had pulled the empty beer bottles down off a shelf and was happily rolling them around the floor. At least I thought they'd been emptied before I left; I didn't think he was opening twist tops and drinking the beer yet. (I did wonder if that would be coming in the next week.) Later, I came down to give him supper, and was relieved at first to see the kitchen looked unchanged. But then I spotted the little bits of plastic scattered all around the floor, and suddenly realized the loaf of bread that had been in the centre of the peninsula, wrapped in plastic, was completely gone. Not a crumb left, and to no one's surprise, Rui wasn't very hungry for his dinner. Empty beer bottles, and eating family food that wasn't his: what could be more typical of an adolescent? I was starting to rethink my earlier sense of enjoyment over his independence.

Another teenage behaviour he started was experimenting with not following instructions. Two weeks earlier if I gave him a boundary ("Rui, kitchen, wait!") he would lie down in there and wait to be released. But suddenly things changed; he might do that, or he might ignore the command, and snap at my hand or leg as he followed me back into the living room. If I turned to take him back into the kitchen, he would dash ahead of me, and then look up as if to say, "See? Here I am just as you wanted. What's your problem, dude?" Then he'd follow me back into the living room. Clearly he knew what he should do, but didn't feel he always had to do it.

Teenagers also push boundaries, and I remembered a few confrontations I couldn't solve in the classroom. ("Student, office, wait!") With Rui I would try the boundary a few more times, and if he wouldn't follow it, he got a "time-out" with the crate door closed till he became more malleable. I hated to lock him up, but disliked the idea of having a dog who chose when he was going to obey rules even more. I had hated sending students to the office—it always felt like a personal failure—but sometimes it had been the best of the bad alternatives.

It wasn't all confrontation; much of the time Rui was very affectionate and friendly. After our walk and conflict, I really wanted an afternoon nap. So I lay down on the living room couch, and let Rui into the room, carefully taking off my glasses and putting them on the window sill behind the couch, safely out of his way. He came over and stared at my face intently; it was the first time he'd seen me without glasses. (I put them on first thing in the morning, and take them off last thing at night.) Then he gently and lovingly licked my face, before jumping up on the couch. He looked around, saw the glasses on the window sill, picked them up (he's inherited a retriever's soft mouth), and carefully put them down next to me.

So the next day, Diana and I redid the kitchen. All the middle shelves were filled with indestructible items. The peninsula top was empty, and the drawers had a vertical pole through their handles preventing them from being pulled open. I found an even more hideous cinnamon shaker at Value Village for seventy cents. It was made out of thick wood, so even if Rui did get it, it would take him a while to chew through. Diana and I made a twenty-five cent bet as to whether Rui would ever figure out how to open the fridge door. I thought he would, but wouldn't be unhappy if I lost. The next morning I woke up wondering what new skill Rui would learn this day. Whatever happened next, it wouldn't be either expected or dull. That was part of the joy of working with teens, whether they were of the two-legged or four-legged variety. It was good to know all the creative chaos hadn't left my life; Eris was still around.

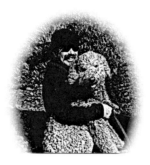

15. Our Own Happiness

*"Your own happiness doesn't
necessarily teach you what you want to know."*

The Who, *Now I'm a Farmer*

A few weeks later I was walking with Rui along one of our neighbourhood's back alleys, that web of shadowy subtext to the official streets that make it onto the maps. As I watched him, I thought about the real world and the gap between it and its shadowy subtext, the world of our desires. What might Rui have desired in his perfect life? There would be a lot of exploring; he had started to walk along half the time with his nose an inch above the ground, clearly following various scents holding fascinating information. His perfect world would have had a lot of food in it, real meat that needed to be gnawed off bones rather than little brown pellets with a vague relationship with meat somewhere way back in their industrial history. And there would have been lots of friendly dogs to play with, an endless parade of squeaky toys to be destroyed, and no leashes.

But most of all in Rui's perfect world, Diana or I would have been with him all the time, because we were his pack. Sadly, what happened to him in the real world was after we came in from a walk, I dried his feet, took off my coat and boots, and went off to do work, leaving him alone in the kitchen. While he was walked twice a day for about two hours by me or by Diana, and we played with him for at least another hour in the evening, he still spent a lot of time alone in the kitchen with his box of chew toys, his bowl of water, and not much else. And of course, that was why we sometimes came home to find various things chewed up and torn apart – he was a smart animal, and he was bored.

But he had to settle for what he got and as a city dog's life went, I could tell myself it was probably pretty good. Had Rui gone to his original about-to-be owners, who were living on the 22nd floor of a condominium, his life would have been even more limited. Their decision not to get him was probably a happy one for them, for us, and most of all for Rui. I was happier living with him, despite the occasional spikes of kitchen chaos, and the imposition of a sterner structural discipline on my day than I was used to.

But even though I could choose the shape of my life in a way he couldn't, I found myself wrestling with the question of where my deepest desire lay. I got to check my emails, socialize with friends, and spend as much time with Rui as I liked. I was in the rare and enviable position of not having to work to earn money, thanks to 32 years of deposits in the teachers' retirement plan. I could eat what I wanted (though it was increasing obvious even to me that it wasn't really a good idea to eat as much as I wanted.) I lived with a woman I dearly loved, who loved me, and we had learned and continued to learn to nourish and support each other through the dark times. So why wasn't all that enough?

I knew that more material things – a mid-life crisis sports-car? – wouldn't make me happier. But perhaps there was a way of living involving more urgency, more pressure, more of a sense I was making a difference. Teaching had some aspects of that, but too much of the urgency and pressure (*How can I get all these exams marked by the due date for final marks?*) was superficial, served no real purpose other than bureaucratic. So wherever my future lay, it wasn't in my past. Been there, done that, got the pension. I had learned what I needed to from teaching high school.

And what was it I wanted to know? How to raise a puppy so he became a well-mannered and happy dog, and I was learning that by doing it. As the Taoist saying advises, I was making the road by walking on it. Learning to be more creative and compassionate was another goal, and Rui was doing his part in helping me towards that. I needed a new social group, and though I didn't fully know it yet, my fellow dog-walkers in High Park were to become part of the solution there.

One difficulty in opening a new future lay in the commitments of the present. My cup had to have some empty space before anything could be poured into it. After I'd left high school teaching, I had taken on everything I could, so as to have things to do. Between teaching online, writing, and volunteering in various groups, the quantity of my obligations was impressive. But my life still felt like a jigsaw puzzle, and I couldn't find the piece that finished it because I couldn't see the completed image and didn't know the shape of the empty space. And without knowing either of those, how could I look at all the possible pieces strewn on the table and say, "Yes, this is the piece I need?"

A close friend said to me, "You have been de-centered," and that carried a ring of truth. Teaching had formed the centre of my work life for so many years that to shift my identity from "I am a high school teacher" to something new was a process I was going through, not yet a place at which I had arrived. But it was time to go and feed Rui, who hadn't had his supper yet and had been waiting patiently. Whatever shadowy sub-textual future was waiting for me to inhabit it, simple duties of feeding and walking the pup were going to be part of it. As the Zen proverb said, "Before enlightenment: chop wood, carry water. After enlightenment: chop wood, carry water." Rui was slowly teaching me to remain more grounded, which was one of the lessons I seemed to need to learn continually.

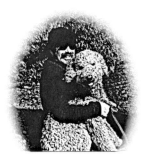

16. The Powder Hound

"Set my compass north
I got winter in my blood"

The Band, *Acadian Driftwood*

It was about two years ago, just as I was leaving teaching, when I decided I needed to regain my childhood joy in winter, which had once been my favourite season. I remembered jumping into huge drifts and pouring snow over my friends' heads, and having them do the same to me. My parents had always skied, from their childhoods into their eighties. My brother and I had each started at three years old. Many of my most ecstatic physical memories were of skiing, at Aspen, at Val D'Isère, at Mont Ste Anne. In the Montreal of my childhood, snowblowers would cruise the streets after a winter storm, aiming their movable guns away from driveways. That produced three metre mounds of firmly packed snow at driveway edges which we could hollow out into caves complete with spiralling passages or turreted forts to defend in our endless snowball fights.

But somewhere that joy had slipped away. Perhaps it had gradually melted when I had moved to Ontario from Québec, and my winters became torpid and slushy rather than crisp and clear. Gradually winter had become a time for staying indoors, for waiting for the cold to pass. To try and regain that joy in cold, I started going for long winter walks, and bought an annual season pass to Horseshoe Valley, a local ski hill offering convenience and cheap cost, though it truly is a valley rather than a mountain. But while I thought I was making good progress in regaining my pleasure in Canadian winters, compared to Rui I was no more than a mere snowbird (a local term of contempt for wimpy Canuks who flee freezing flakes to fry in Floridian fetor).

This was partially because Rui's curly coat trapped air so well, and made him immune to such cold as Toronto winters had. We walked for two hours every day, and in the –15º C. temperatures we had for a week, he showed no signs of being cold. I never saw him shiver, even when his muzzle was covered with icicles. One day it was –30º and I thought that was the day we'd see how much cold he could bear, but somewhere on the far side of the two hour mark, it was me who wanted to come in, to Rui's regret.

So having a dog changed the question about what lay on the other side of the window pane from "Do I really want to go outside in weather like this?" to "What do I need to wear to go out in this weather?" I would repeat to myself the fine saying by Ranulph Fiennes, an intrepid British polar explorer who climbed Everest at age 65, that there's no such thing as bad weather, there's only inappropriate clothing. On the prow of the canoe that hung in my garage I had once put a picture of Queen Victoria, over her words (to Gladstone, during the war in Crimea), "We are not interested in the possibilities of defeat." Similarly, Rui was imperiously disinterested in the possibilities of not having a walk. When we went out, he'd always choose the route through the deepest snow. If we came to a particularly deep drift, he'd plunge his head into it, and root around happily. He showed a clear preference for virgin snow over something already tracked, and would always try to dive into it. When the snow was under 30 centimetres deep and only came up to his body, he'd wade through it, but if it was deeper, he had a spectacular leaping motion I'd never seen in dogs, one that looked like a tawny jack-rabbit, with both his front paws and back paws moving together as he leapt through the drifts.

One day we had some freezing rain after 30 centimetres of snow which resulted in a thin ice crust with powder beneath it. I was walking down the centre of the back alleys, avoiding the deeper drifts along the edges. Rui, who always chose to walk on snow rather than pavement, was delighted to walk on the unbroken ice so it would crack beneath his paws. He'd eagerly head across the alley if he spotted an unmarked patch of snow on the other side, and proudly stomp through the ice with his high stepping poodle gait, leaving his paw prints happily behind.

If Diana or I were shovelling the walk, he wanted us to throw shovelfuls of snow over him, while he barked happily and snapped at the snow in the air. It was absolutely clear this was his idea of a good time, because he'd race over to me and stand waiting for snow to be thrown at him. I knew that if he had opposable thumbs, we'd have been dodging snowballs continually. Once, in a fenced park, an Asian girl of about ten was admiring him from the other side of the fence, and pretending to throw snow at him. I encouraged her to follow through, and for the next five minutes, Rui pushed up against the chain links while she gleefully dumped armfuls of powder over him.

Mom called him a "powder hound", the traditional name for skiers who seek out fresh powder, and it certainly fit. During our walks we were amused to pass toy dogs shivering beneath their patterned woollen coats and tap-dancing in their little booties. His autumnal grass seizures became snow seizures, as he squirmed ecstatically on his back, leaving snow puppies that reminded me of the snow angels I had made as a child. One day I was wrestling Rui in a park, pinned him down, and started pouring snow over his head (as I had done and received in my childhood). He loved it, trying to swallow as much of the snow as he could. I scraped as much as

I could into a pile by his nose, and he immediately stuck his head into it.

I noticed in winter there were fewer people in parks with their dogs, which made me wonder whether it was the dogs or the owners who didn't like the snow and ice, or their owners. But Lady Fortune clearly smiled on us; when Diana and I were choosing a breed, we had never thought about their tolerance for snow and cold. What luck to have stumbled onto a snow puppy who could help me trek back into my childhood winter delights.

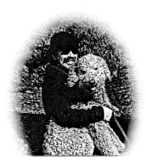

17. Rui Roams the House

"Throw my ticket out the window,
Throw my suitcase out there, too,
Throw my troubles out the door,
I don't need them any more
'Cause tonight I'll be staying here with you."

Bob Dylan, *Tonight I'll Be Staying Here With You.*

M y dear friend Gabe came over to visit me. As soon as he entered the house Rui bounded up to him and wriggled ecstatically, and then leapt up on him so as to be able to lick him better. I pulled Rui down, eventually got him to sit, and shook my head apologetically. "Sometimes I think I'm doing a really good job with Rui, and sometimes I feel like an utter failure."

Gabe, a father, just smiled. "Welcome to parenthood."

It had been four and a half months since Rui had come into our lives, which meant he was just over six months old. And some things had improved at home. Rui had feared longer staircases when he was younger. Four or five steps, such as those at the front or back door, never presented a problem, but the longer and steeper stairs that lead up or down from the main floor were frightening to him. Diana and I would stand upstairs and implore him to come up and join us. But he'd only gaze up, whimper a few times, and then skulk away rather than continue to be humiliated. I sympathized with that behaviour; as a teenager, I'd stopped going to high school dances for similar reasons.

Suzanne taught us to just take his leash and walk up the stairs, and he'd (perforce) follow. We did that a few times to be sure it worked for us as well as it had for her, but then thought how until Rui stopped chewing on everything we weren't sure we really wanted him upstairs. After the earlier incidents with the tea candles, and the plastic bags, Rui had to spend all day in the kitchen unless he was being walked or we were downstairs to supervise him in the living and dining rooms. It had seemed too dangerous to our possessions, and to him, to let him free in rooms with fine rugs and extension cords. I even joked I could see a time ahead when we'd look back to his being marooned on the first floor as a golden era when the upstairs and basement were safe. I was completely wrong.

The change happened while I was spending a happy ten days in Vancouver with David and his family. During that time Diana chose to create art out at home, rather than going over to her studio. That way she could walk, feed, and be around Rui. She decided to follow the advice given in the Monks' "The Art of Raising a Puppy" and try keeping him near even when she was upstairs at the computer. And after I returned, I followed her example because so much changed when he got to be upstairs with me. Even though I wasn't playing, being near me calmed him. He knew he wasn't missing out on the action, and he'd chew one of his toys, or sleep peacefully at my feet. Sometimes he'd go downstairs for a drink of water or to get a different toy, but he would always return upstairs pretty quickly.

And as always, change cut both ways. Because he was spending more time with me, and much of that time he wasn't my primary focus, Rui became more and more a companion rather than a duty. He had always been a very enjoyable and much loved duty, but usually our shared time was spent walking together, or in feeding, grooming or play. Now he was suddenly sharing the house, and I felt even closer to him. Part of that was because his freedom to wander around made him less bored and better behaved. Part of it was what I would later come to recognize as the beginning of a change to a more egalitarian relationship, one in which it wasn't my job to correct his behaviour continuously.

Like so many of the things I'd learned, this seemed so obvious in retrospect. In my classroom I had eliminated the traditional school ritual of requiring students to put their hands up to get official permission before they could go to the bathroom. If they needed to, they just got up and left. If they went too often, or were gone for too long, the privilege was revoked. But by not clinging to a fairly pointless piece of authority, a whole area of conflict disappeared. So with Rui: when we allowed him to be with us, a lot of the destructive bored behaviour we'd been fighting vanished. Lao-Tse, the founder of Taoism, wrote that the more prohibitions you have, the less virtuous people will be. Apparently Taoism works for dogs as well.

The success of keeping Rui near us during the day made us rethink continuing to shut him in the kitchen at night. The Monks' other book, "How to Be Your Dog's Best Friend" argued strongly against keeping him apart. So we tried having Rui in the bedroom at night, but while he would come upstairs with us, he preferred sleeping downstairs. About three or four hours after going to sleep we'd hear him pawing at the closed bedroom door, and one of us would sleepily let him out. (Eventually, we figured out it was easier just to leave the door open.) He'd wander downstairs, and in the morning we'd find him in either of his two favourite sleeping spots, in his crate or on the living room couch. (He had won that battle.) He'd rub against us sleepily, but we got up earlier than he did, and he wasn't ready to play or even to eat yet. Rui enjoyed waking up slowly. Over the next few months these patterns evolved and became a mix of what we all wanted, not just Diana and my rules. It was clear everything worked better when Rui got to have some say in how things went.

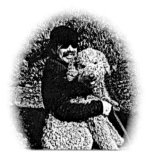

18. THE SHADOW OF THE DOG

"You're the same
You're the same
You're the same kind of bad as me"

Tom Waits *Bad as Me*

A rchetypal stories and myths serve as templates through which we align our own stories to universal patterns. That's why it's worth studying mythology (of which religion is a subset): not because of its historical truth or falsity, but because of the psychological truths embedded in it. Watching Rui grow, I saw some classic myths in his behaviour. Or more accurately, some of my projections onto him fitted mythical patterns, which is not all that surprising. Mythical patterns are how we see the world.

A simple example: Rui, having finally solved the mystery of stairs, came into our bedroom one morning where he was struck by his own reflection in the floor length mirror. He went over to the mirror and stared, then came closer, and tried to lick the handsome dog he saw there. Fortunately the only results were tongue marks at Rui-height on the mirror, unlike Narcissus, who thought himself so beautiful he drowned trying to embrace his own reflection in the mirror of a pool.

A sadder myth was our contemporary version of the dog who cried wolf. Back when Rui had spent the nights in his crate in the kitchen, he generally slept the night through, but from time to time he would start barking. At first Diana or I would get up, go downstairs, check that his mini-water bowl was filled, take him outside to relieve himself. But invariably, nothing happened. He just wanted to play, or to be let out. So we started ignoring his plaintive barks, and in the morning everything was just fine.

My first night back from Vancouver, I got to bed around midnight only to be awakened at 2 a.m. by prolonged barking. Diana and I looked at each other; I had taken him out before closing the crate and filled his water bowl. We ignored the hour of barking, and eventually it stopped. At 6 a.m. Diana got up; I hoped to sleep for another hour but was summoned to see the dog, his crate and the surrounding kitchen floor all covered with the diarrhea he had tried to warn us was coming. (The floor had gotten it when he had backed his bum against the mesh of the cage; the poor guy was doing the best he could not to soil his den.)

Did Rui learn not to bark when he didn't really need attention? I doubted it; archetypes are patterns that repeat through time, and he lived in the immediate world. But did Peter and Diana learn their lesson to not prejudge his barking? No shit....

After his stair breakthrough, Rui had roamed the house, following Diana and me. It was a joy to have him with us, even if he hadn't completely figured out yet how to relax. We excited him, so he wanted to play or to climb on us. Napping could be done in those boring times when he was alone. But it seemed as though we'd moved to a higher level of companionship. Maybe, I thought, our troubles are over. And of course I continually projected my canine archetypes onto him, images of Lassie, Rin-Tin-Tin, Buck, and all the faithful, heroic and unfailingly affectionate dogs of my youth. I kept imagining one more lesson or the next walk would transform him into a wise and infallible companion who never needed to be reprimanded, and would only run off when he needed to tell Diana I had once again fallen down the well.

But then came a darker archetype with which I was to wrestle for a long time. I saw in (or projected onto) Rui the increasing emergence of a shadow side, perhaps an evil Muttster Hyde behind the usual friendliness of Doggy Jekyll. Just as in the Robert Louis Stevenson story where the gentle kind doctor would suddenly transform into a monster of evil, Rui seemed to suddenly shift between two separate personalities.

This new trouble appeared on our walks. The earlier episodes of leash biting suddenly evolved into attacks on the leash holder. He'd turn from a loveable – albeit independent minded – companion into an angry dog, growling, leaping and snapping at our hands or arms. Diana came home after one such walk saying it was the first time she'd ever been scared of him. The next day I knew what she meant, even if my reaction was fight rather than flight. It was as though Rui were attacking me. These incidents happened in particular when he wanted something we weren't giving him: a chance to socialize with another person or dog, but anything could trigger an episode, leash corrections, or asking him to sit before crossing a street. And it triggered my anger again, as I felt I had to establish my Alpha role. As Rui changed, so my own compassionate Dr. Jekyll would suddenly be displaced by the evil Mr. Hyde.

We developed some moderately functional ways of dealing with the problem. Forcing him to lie down by standing on his chain, and waiting till his mood changed was the most reliable. I was hugely upset this was happening and wrote a desperate letter to Suzanne, our trainer, but there was no response. Perhaps it was puberty and testosterone kicking in? He was also starting to hump us on any occasion he could, and to that at least we knew the solution. One sad morning (for him at least) he went in for his neutering operation, and I picked him up in the afternoon together with a hefty bill. This was again not covered by the insurance as it was elective surgery, at least from our perspective if not Rui's. As well, we were given a set of instructions that seemed increasingly irrelevant. No exercise for a week to ten days? Don't worry if he doesn't eat for a few days, or drink for a day? The next morning Rui was enthusiastic, thirsty, very hungry, and on a long walk he attacked me with more ferocity than I'd ever seen. The good news was he was recovering well. The bad news was nothing much seemed changed, though he gradually humped less. How to deal with Muttster Hyde?

I returned to "How To Be Your Dog's Best Friend", the book by the Monks of New Skete, which had a long session on discipline. Shaking him by the scruff of the neck seemed to be the most promising recommendation. Bringing my face right up to his, and saying, "Rui! No!" while shaking him seemed to puzzle him (Why are you mad at me?) and abash him. Generally, he'd switch back into Doggy Jekyll. For a day or two, I was optimistic.

Suzanne finally returned my call, saying it was all normal seven month puppy behaviour for an assertive dog. She reassured me we didn't have a demon dog. But she also said I should spend less time with him, not more as the Monks say. (On most issues they had been in complete agreement, so that difference was interesting in itself.) She said the biting was normal teenage behaviour. Certainly I saw analogous behaviour among my erstwhile students: self-centred, utterly loveable and affectionate one moment, furiously rebellious the next (though I never had one try to bite me). And a teenage rebellion thesis fitted well with a view that what was really going on was Rui wanted to be in charge of his life, not have us making rules he had to obey. Aside from less time with Rui (we decided we were unwilling to follow that), she recommended lots of long stay down time, something the Monks also counselled. So I tried getting him to lie down, to sit more, and he was generally his affectionate Doggy Jekyll self. But when we had a walk coming up, I still worried at what moment Muttster Hyde might suddenly spring out at me. And often he did.

And that became my shadow dog, the fear that despite all our training efforts there was a Bad Dog in Rui who could never be tamed. Again, I was haunted by Red Wull, a top sheep-herder by day but a pathological sheep-killer at night. With teenagers in conflict, I could always talk to them and however hostile they were, we could reduce the conflict to an objective external difference: if you do (or don't do) these things, I can't have you in the class. But Rui was never big on meaningful discussions, and I became less sure how much of what I saw as his essential nature was only my projection. What lay behind that furry face? And maybe it wasn't consistent: maybe he was just an irreparable mixture of good and bad, like the two-legged ones.

At the beginning of my career, I had believed there were a set of ways to teach, and once I learned them, I'd be a teacher. It took a while to understand I had to find my own way to teach, as the Maths teacher in Brixton had told me, and it took longer than that for me to realize there was no one way to teach everyone. Each student was unique. I've always wanted – perhaps we all have – an infallible guide who'll reveal the right thing to do. When I went into therapy, what I really wanted was for my therapist to hear my problems, then give me the magical answer, after which everything would work. And part of maturing has been learning, over and over, that there's no such thing. The fine Zen Buddhist saying, "If you meet the Buddha on the road, kill him," warns us that setting up anyone as infallible is an idolatrous mistake. So having the Monks and Suzanne in disagreement was useful. I had to start letting go of their authority, and start to find my own way through. But what way was that? What was needed when my dog leapt at me, snapping and growling? Was there something I was doing wrong? Was it something wrong with him? I knew the questions always came before the answers, but being between them was a hard and fearful place.

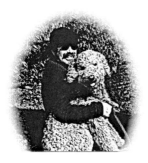

19. Mature for His Age

"Little round planet
In a big universe
Sometimes it looks blessed
Sometimes it looks cursed
Depends on what you look at, obviously
But even more it depends on the way that you see"

Bruce Cockburn *Child of the Wind*

s winter ended, the sun was melting the last of the snow and revealing the buried garbage beneath, like a therapist uncovering material that has been repressed or denied. It felt to me as though things were getting worse with Rui at home. He certainly was happy to be with me as much as possible through the day. But that was because he wanted to play. When I didn't want to, he got feisty. There was the day I was desperately trying to get an ad designed before the Tikkun Toronto meeting for which it was promised. Suddenly my computer froze. Not just the program, but the whole system: neither typing nor any mouse movement would produce the slightest response. I always assure my PC owning friends that on a Mac this never happens...and then I realized:

Rui was at my feet and had smoothly bitten through the cable that connects the computer and keyboard. I took him downstairs and saw more bits of cable. He'd warmed up by chewing through the IKEA wire protection tube, and then devoured the stereo cable inside that fed the right living room speaker. Fortunately, he'd left the 110 volt power line for the lamp untouched; it was in the same tube, adjacent to the stereo cable.

I bought a new usb cable for the computer. (The salesman looked puzzled when asked if any of their cables were guaranteed dog proof.) I rewired the stereo and put more tube around all the cables soaking it in "Sour Apple", a spray advertised to repel dogs. I locked Rui back in the kitchen for awhile, and later came downstairs to find he'd managed to tear off the moldings surrounding the kitchen door, a feat I wouldn't have thought possible for a dog. Was doggy Hyde starting to manifest in the house? It was beginning to look as though I should look into renting him to a demolition company.

Outside the house, the problems continued with Rui's leaping and biting on walks. His bites weren't full out attacks, but they were nips that hurt, and I was sure they weren't what a well trained dog should do. I began dreading walks, and kept trying different ways to get Rui to stop these behaviours. Grabbing his collar, and putting him immediately into a "down" was what Suzanne recommended, but he'd often start leaping again as soon as he was released. I tried guilt (hey, it worked on me when I was a kid!), yelling "Ouch!" when he leapt up. I tried being gentle and getting him to sit, and petting him. All of these methods worked some of the time, but not others.

And there were other problems. Rui showed far more interest in objects on the ground, and in following up smells I couldn't guess at than in heeling as I wanted. I was getting desperate: had we been dealt a Bad Dog in the poker game of fate? And what would we do if that were the case? Looking at Rui, I was starting to see a bad dog, an uncontrolled animal who might attack at any moment. That projection of my own uncertainty onto him of course didn't feel like a projection; it felt like an accurate expectation of what was going to happen, just as projections always feel.

Later I would remember the classic educational study in which half an incoming Grade nine class, chosen at random, are identified to their teachers as gifted students expected to make major educational gains in the coming year. And– wonderful to relate– at the end of that year, the identified group had indeed improved much more than the other half. The two groups were in fact academically equal, but the teachers' expectations trumped reality.

Fortunately it was time for Rui and I to have our next lesson with Suzanne, who came ready to deal with both our problems. Although eagerly anticipating this day, I did feel like the kid who never practices his piano lessons until the day before the next lesson. Suzanne had already given me many fine techniques that I should have been practicing regularly with Rui, and I felt guilty over how many times it was easier to close a door rather than give a boundary and spend the next twenty minutes repeating it, or the times he was allowed to meander over people's front lawns rather than being pressed to heel. But I needed Suzanne's insights not only because she was a professional trainer, but because she had started her career working with "challenging" dogs.

So when Rui greeted Suzanne's arrival with too much enthusiasm, leaping up happily and trying to lick her face, I was pleased. A clear demonstration of the problem! But he calmed down, and then we all went for a walk. Suzanne taught me a new method of getting him to heel, using two leashes. The second was looser, and dragged on the ground. If he surged ahead, I would step on it, and he would be forced to stop. After a while he walked placidly at my side. It was, of course, a Doggy Jekyll day, so he was well behaved. He sat placidly on a busy Bloor West sidewalk and let people walk past without trying to lunge at them. And when we got home, Suzanne said he was really a wonderful dog, and "very mature for his age". He just needed more challenges.

I was hugely pleased to hear this; "very mature for his age" made me think of many other report card phrases that might apply to

Rui. He plays well with others. He's very good at resting. He's gloriously good-natured, most of the time. And he just needed more challenges. So the next day Diana and I took him for a long car ride (he behaved well) to a conservation area about an hour north of Toronto. There I put him on a loose leash and wandered through dense woods, to see if he would follow me or get tangled by choosing alternative routes. He passed...never getting hooked. We went to a lake, where he waded in up to his stomach, and looked as though he were considering taking his first swim. (Lots of algae: I discouraged him.) He explored the lake shore till he found the conservation authority's water intake pipe, on which he immediately began to chew. (When I told him I didn't think that was very mature behaviour, he stopped.) He happily devoured a long dead mouse he found, which Diana pointed out is mature in terms of wolves and hunting behaviour.

Monday was a sunny warm spring day, so I took Rui for two long walks. Both times he was well behaved on leash. At Dufferin Grove park we met a half dozen other dogs, and I let him off: with other dogs around he wouldn't roam. I called him back to me several times, and he came running each time to be greeted with treats and enthusiasm. I tried having him sit and stay on Bloor and although there were plastic bags blowing by, people walking past, and cars driving by endlessly he peacefully stayed in his position until released. Later we sat on the front porch and watched the thunderstorm roll through; he was interested in lightning, but pleasingly undisturbed by thunder. He clearly was a mature dog; I didn't know how I could have missed it. It's very fortunate Suzanne pointed it out to me.

The Sufis have a saying, "When the thief looks at the wise man, all he sees are his pockets." That's because that's what he's looking for. So once I was able to look for Rui's maturity, I started to see it a lot more. Yes, the biting and leaping was a problem. But the real problem, the shadowy projection of Muttster Hyde onto Rui was a problem that lay at the other end of the leash, even if I hadn't fully realized it yet.

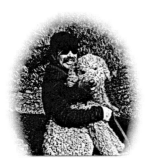

20. So Much Love

"I can hardly wait
To see you come of age
But I guess we'll both just have to be patient
'Cause it's a long way to go
A hard row to hoe
Yes it's a long way to go
But in the meantime
Before you cross the street
Take my hand
Life is what happens to you
While you're busy making other plans"

John Lennon *Beautiful Boy*

Once it had been pointed out to me that Rui was mature, I began to appreciate who he was a bit more, and worry about changing him a bit less. He was eight months old, which meant he'd been living with us for half a year. Half a year! It seemed yesterday we had brought home a cute little three kilogram puppy who had cried through much of the first night. Now we had a 25 kilogram beast who happily leapt onto my stomach while I dozed on the couch, and seemed surprised at my violent reaction when his paw landed on my crotch. I didn't think he was taking a deliberate revenge for our neutering him a month earlier.

There was a continual fascination in seeing his personality emerge. Never having lived with a growing puppy, I was unsure how many of his characteristics were probably standard doggy behaviour (never being too full for a treat, and always being convinced what we're eating is more interesting than what he was given. This latter belief was, of course, quite accurate.) He had the traditional Labrador energy; the Monks' guide book said to give him enough of a walk to tire him out twice a day, but we'd come to realize even with cunningly spaced handovers both Diana and I would be exhausted long before Rui would. It was when he hadn't had enough exercise he was most likely to be nippy and ignore boundaries; when tired, Rui was much better behaved (which, curiously, was just the opposite of how I was). Other dogs were the only thing that could exhaust him, so we frequented off-leash dog parks where both of us could socialize with our respective species.

That meant we were learning more about other dogs, as well as our own. But he still seemed individual. His dominant characteristic was affection. This was particularly so with Diana and I, of course: we were his pack. He'd follow us upstairs and downstairs, insatiably curious about what we were doing. One day he stood intently watching me in the jacuzzi, possibly debating whether to jump in. When I got out, he started enthusiastically licking me dry, but sadly accepted my preference for a towel. He had learned when I was at the computer my focus was off him, so he would nudge my mouse hand with his nose so I had to pay attention to him. (This resulted in very bad training on my part: all teachers agree that you should never give positive reinforcement, like laughing or hugging, for negative behaviour.)

Not everyone found his doggy persona appealing, of course. One morning I encountered a dog owner who studied Rui carefully, and then asked what breed he was. I explained, and the owner responded that his own dog was 100% poodle, (emphasis on the

100%, clearly implying that Rui was a lesser creature at a mere 62.5% poodle.) He said that he'd never met a labradoodle who wasn't goofy, though he allowed that as Rui was only a puppy he was still permitted to be that way. I was amused at the time, but thinking about it later was struck by the extent to which my goofy dog made me happy. Yes, he ran into an amazing number of things every day, but that was because his utter joy in doing whatever he was doing (chasing a ball) lead him to crash into the wall he hadn't noticed. I watched him in High Park intently tracing a scent with his nose to the ground, and walking right into the edge of a picnic table. He always retained his puppyish inner joy that manifested in spectacular forward somersaults, followed by lying on his back wriggling happily and waving all four limbs in the air in a grass seizure. It was goofy, but also utterly joyful and uninhibited. I supposed some people would find the Dalai Lama too goofy for their tastes too.

It was only on walks with Diana or me that Muttster Hyde would come out; we never saw any other aggression in him. We could take whatever he was chewing on away from him, and while he might try and keep it (the dead mouse he found had a particular appeal) he wouldn't growl or snap at us. Other visiting dogs were welcome to chew his favourite bone, or play with whatever toy they want. The one exception was small squeaky toys, which he would never surrender, for food, for praise, or under command.

But while Rui wasn't possessive, he had developed a sense of territoriality, a sense that the pack's house was something he needed to protect. He was lying with Diana on the couch one day when he suddenly started barking. This was unusual...he's such a quiet dog that sometimes two or three days will go by without a single bark. Looking out from the window, Diana saw someone walking across our front lawn. Two days later, she left the first load of groceries outside the back door rather than bringing them in. Again, Rui barked, hearing someone outside on our property. So it appeared we'd gotten ourselves a watchdog to protect the house. If someone did try to break and enter on some dark and stormy night, they might be frightened to hear a big dog barking, and if not, he'd leap on them and lick them to death when they did get in.

The territoriality also extended to a new sense of our back or front yard as inappropriate places to pee. We religiously took him out last thing at night before putting him into his crate, but he almost never used that opportunity. Instead he'd stand in the back yard, head up in the air, nose twitching, as he intently took in the scents, light-years beyond my perception, that clearly communicated a fascinating story to him. Fortunately, he had amazing bladder control, so after his afternoon walk around three or four, he'd not pee again until his morning walk at eight. Diana and I both envied him that ability.

This new sense led to perhaps the only time I'd ever heard Rui growl seriously. He had growled during our tugs of war, or while rolling over in play fight with another dog at Bickford Park, but it had always been very clear it was play. But this was serious to him. I was lying on the bed reading a fine Jonathan Lethem novel when Rui wandered in to see what I was doing. Suddenly he noticed the curtains billowing with the wind. He looked at them, backed up a few feet (no sense in taking chances) and started growling from deep in his chest. I saw what his concern was, finally stopped laughing, and went over and pulled the curtains out, so he could see that they were just cloth. He came over when I called him, saw what they were, and immediately got this, "Yeah, I knew they were cloth all along. OMG, you didn't really think I was serious did you?" look on his face. Then he pointedly ignored the curtains for the rest of the evening.

He was universally affectionate with other dogs, ranging from the 80 kilogram mastiff he tried to leap on (fortunately it was muzzled, as it clearly was not amused, as the owner desperately hanging on to its steel-link chain made clear) to tiny toy puppies before whom he'll roll over and wave his paws enticingly, hoping to lure them into play. He had a doodle way of initiating play in which he batted the other dog with his paw. If that didn't work, Rui would try different techniques until he found one that did, or until the dog wandered off, leaving him bereft.

He was also unusually sociable with people. When we'd arrive at a dog park, he'd often go and greet the owners before saying hello to their dogs. On walks Rui always liked to stop and lick a passersby when allowed to. He was much more excited when a stranger came in than when Diana or I came home. We'd get a tail wag and wriggle; they got the full leap up ecstasy of puppy enthusiasm. It was about this time I was walking him and we passed a teenager (punk hair, piercings, leather) listening to her iPod. It made me think how much I missed the contact with teens I had while teaching. But then she saw Rui, paused her iPod and asked if she could pet him. She rubbed him; he wriggled ecstatically and licked her hand and then she turned to me and said in amazement, "So much love!" It was a glorious miracle, and such a joy to live with.

Rui was increasingly delightful. When a dog doesn't behave it's obviously either because he doesn't want to, or because he doesn't understand what's wanted. With Rui it was always the first; he wouldn't lie down on command, for example, unless there was a treat involved. Then he was down in a flash. I knew I was probably spoiling him with too much affection, but he was spoiling me the same way, so it felt okay. And if it weren't, I didn't really care. I was forming a relationship with this strange non-human based on how we could all make it work, rather than clutching the full list of correct Good Canine Citizenship traits and forcing him to fit that mold. Rui was still teaching me to get out of my head space, and more into my emotions and body. That felt a bit scary, as I'd always been more comfortable in my head. But if I were going to engage with him, it couldn't be intellectually. He just wasn't going to go there.

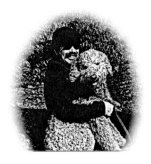

21. CHANGES

"Where have they gone our little ones little ones
Where have they gone our children our own
Turn around and they're young turn around and they're old
Turn around and they've gone and we've no one to hold"

Charlie Louvin *Turn Around*

Time passes imperceptibly, and its changes are always easier to see from a distance: the friend we hadn't seen for a decade looked so different when we met; the parents we returned to after two years had aged dramatically, while our non-prodigal sibling who stayed at home didn't see any changes at all. We have created artificial markers to mark times' changes, birthdays, rites of passage, borders to tell us we're entering or leaving one country, even if the land on this side of the border is utterly indistinguishable from that on the other. But change still accrues as the only constant in people's lives, and in a dog's.

It seemed unlikely Rui's changes happened during the two weeks Diana was away with her mother, or the week I was away in Quebec for my annual Victoria Day bacchanal. Our trips overlapped, so for four days Rui was staying with a friend (of ours, though later of his). More likely our being away just helped us to see them. At first I wondered if the changes were cosmetic: his first hair cut left him looking less like a canine Rastafarian, and more like a poodle. Was it just my continuing internalizing of Suzanne's observation on his maturity? But the facts seemed to be there: at nine months our puppy was definitely getting more mature. He certainly was still a puppy (hugely enthusiastic, high energy, full of amusing clumsiness) but we could see the adult dog emerging. This was hugely reassuring, and made his lapses much more bearable, and perhaps even endearing.

Of course the changes related to Rui were happening in us as well. Diana had warned if we got a dog we'd become one of those boring middle-aged couples, who talk (and write) about nothing else. And verily, so it had come to pass. What we most talked about was Rui's motivation, trying to understand his behaviour, or what he was thinking when he did particular things. We did recognize there was more than a touch of anthropomorphism going on. Diana confessed to me sometimes she thought he was just a small boy in a very well tailored fur coat. She reproached me when I proposed yet another indulgence with, "Peter, he's just a dog," to which I responded in mock-horror, "Don't say that!" We had changed from people who could rationally discuss getting a pet, into neurotics who thought of themselves and their dog as a pack.

Rui had become more confident in his world. When we walked the neighbourhood's back alleys, we'd often pass large dogs penned in their back yards. A few months ago he had been frightened by their barking, and the heavy meaty thuds when their bodies hit their restraining fence. He had either tried to get away, or came in close to me, so I could protect him if needed. (I had whispered, "Don't worry, pup; I can take them," as reassurance.) Now he would just face them silently. Was he enjoying their frustration, wondering why they behaved so curiously, or hoping they'd come out to play? I couldn't tell.

We had reached a point at which he could run off leash during walks in parks, as he usually came when he was called. He would first look to see why. If I were on a different path from him, it was a good reason, and he'd immediately run back to follow me. I was clearly the one who knew the direction we were meant to take. If I weren't visible, he'd panic and run frantically back to find me. But if I were in sight, on the same path, and there didn't seem to be a good reason to come, he'd finish investigating whatever scent he was involved with before returning. Gradually Diana and I came to be part of a group of about seven or eight people who met every morning in High Park, at 7 A.M., to walk our dogs. All the dogs were about the same age and size, and while they socialized and explored the park, we would walk and talk and share what was happening in our lives. They became our friends, just as the teachers with whom I'd taught had been, only instead of a bonding over students and their behaviours, we had our dogs and their issues.

For Rui it was squeaky toys. If I threw a squeaky toy of his, he'd retrieve it, bring it back, and sometimes even drop it. But if he had grabbed a squeaky toy belonging to another dog, he'd refuse to give it back, either by staying out of reach, or keeping his jaws clamped on it. The impasse would last until he was back in the car, or at home, which were clearly areas in which we were allowed to take squeaky toys away from him. But when we were out in the doggy world, it was finders keepers. It was embarrassing not to be able to return another dog's toys, but the other dogs were either copophiliac (poop eaters), or occasional chasers of joggers, attackers of dogs who weren't in our pack, rollers in disgusting objects of advanced decay, or disappearers into the bushes who didn't return. Squeaky toys were just one of the quirks.

More and more Rui accepted there were Rules, and Diana and I got to make them. A month previously if I had given him a boundary to keep him out of the kitchen, he might either have mock-snapped at me, then followed me right back into that room, or he might have waited till I was in the kitchen, then slipped his legs over the boundary and entered. If I did nothing, he would move his head in, and gradually the rest would follow. Rui understood intuitively the urban myth of the frog who gets boiled to death when the water is heated because there's never quite enough change to make it hop out. Only in his version, I was the unobservant frog, and he was the heating water, imperceptibly crossing the boundary one small paw at a time. Now, a month later, he placidly accepted boundaries. When he got underfoot while I was cooking, I took him into the dining room, and repeated the magical incantation, "Rui: Dining-room. Wait." He looked at me, then sank down on his fore-legs, and settled into a nap.

I looked at him lying in the dining room, and thought how much, for dogs as for people, the wisdom of maturity resembles being too tired. Without that bouncy puppy energy we could hardly contain, he had become a dog, rather than a force of nature. The change wasn't absolute; there were certainly moments when the old Muttster Hyde came out in full force. When I didn't let him play with three small cute children who were on their way to school, he leapt on my hand and nipped it with such ferocity I overheard one boy asking his father, "Daddy, why is that dog attacking his master?" It was a very good question, and I was sad they were too far away for me to hear the father's response.

So we were not fooled the puppy terrorist had been exterminated and the war on terror won. When I bought Rui a dog-frisbee, it came with a lifetime warranty that if it were ever chewed through, all I had to do for a free replacement was to return the receipt with the shredded corpse of the frisbee. I went upstairs and came down later to find that Rui had pulled the frisbee off the counter where I'd left it, and clearly had been playing with it. It was undamaged, which was good. But he'd also pulled the warranty off the counter and chewed up the address that was my only record of where I was supposed to send the damaged one. Napoleon once wrote about the importance of cutting off your enemy's line of retreat before you engage him, and Rui clearly agreed. The Eris–loving part of me was happy he hadn't yet been reduced to abject obedience, despite my best efforts.

Like me, Rui got bored easily. When Diana and I were on the couch watching a movie or reading, Rui would want to be with us, chewing on one of his toys. But in five or ten minutes he'd jump off the couch, go to the kitchen and his toy box, fish out a tempting item, charge back into the living room with it in his mouth, and leap back up on the couch for the next few minutes. By the end of a good evening there would be half a dozen toys scattered around the couch. I hadn't been able to train him to put them back when he was done with them, but remembered my parents had trouble training me to do that, and Diana sometimes still did. When I looked at my non-Rui day, the same pattern emerged; I would write a bit, then respond to the work my creative writing students had submitted, then surf the web looking for tidbits for my weekly newsletter. Maybe if it was okay for Rui to keep switching between toys, it was okay for me too?

I was starting to accept Rui wasn't going to turn out any more perfect than his master. The Writers' Croft wasn't going to make me as much money as teaching high school had. Tikkunista wasn't going to have thousands of readers waiting every week for the next issue. As a teenager I had believed all my inadequacies would be outgrown with maturity. As the years passed, I had slowly learned that recognizing and working with them was the challenge. Outgrowing them might have to wait for the next lifetime. Those had been hard lessons to accept about myself, but either it was easier to accept about a dog or some of the projection of humanity onto him I was doing was useful. Perhaps it was both.

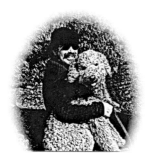

22. Arrival in Gaspé

"Well, I wish I was on some Australian mountain range
Oh, I wish I was on some Australian mountain range
I got no reason to be there, but
I imagine it would be some kind of change."

Bob Dylan *Outlaw Blues*

I've always loved travelling. Maybe I had already acquired the taste for it at three months, when I decided to emigrate from the UK, where I had been born, to settle in Canada. (My parents reached a similar decision at around the same time, I have been told.) As I grew up my family moved between Montreal and Granby, before finally settling in Toronto, where I completed high school. We often travelled, by transcontinental train to see my maternal grandparents in Seattle, or by car to Boston to see my paternal grandmother and her family. After finishing my undergraduate study at MIT in Boston, I worked in England for a year, and travelled around Europe. It was a rare year when I didn't get down to the States at least once, or fly across Canada to see my brother and his family in Vancouver. I had been back to Europe a half dozen times, and had made four trips to south-east Asia, with which I had fallen in love during a lazy sabbatical meander starting in Turkey and six months later reaching Hong Kong.

But now my itchy feet had a ball and chain. How to travel with a puppy? There was the Writers' Croft, my online writing course, to maintain. And the readers of Tikkunista: how would they ever survive without my insights into what had happened in the world that week? But the summer semester had low registration, and Diana and I mulled it over, and decided to spend five weeks on a creative retreat to Gaspé, that remote and beautiful peninsula jutting into the Atlantic Ocean along the southern side of the Gulf of the St Lawrence River. Quebec has always been my favourite part of Canada, and Gaspé was a part of it I hadn't yet explored.

I canceled the summer session of the Writers' Croft, and announced the newsletter would resume in the fall. Perhaps my fear of retirement being an empty time had led me too far in the opposite direction, towards filling all my time with activities? The plan was to let the summer trip be empty, fertile soil allowing for new growth. The world would probably still be waiting when I came back. And while I loved my home and the fullness of my life there, I knew there needed to be a yin, an empty receptive time and space to contrast the yang, to maintain a healthy balance of being with doing. I hoped we could find a place where Diana could paint, I could write, and Rui could enjoy long walks with us through a new countryside. Spending time in a creative retreat together felt like a good plan.

After completing the slow process of asking our friends if any of their friends had friends who had a house for rent in Gaspé (short answer: no), we turned to a high intensity internet search. Success! We found a three week rental in the tiny town of Le Manche d'Épée, ("The Handle of the Sword") and decided the final two weeks would find a place to happen before they came due. We filled our Toyota Echo, with Rui ensconced in the hatchback, the backseat filled with foodstuffs and art/tech equipment, and the $1400 Yakima roof-top cargo carrier (a.k.a. the sky-coffin) stuffed with Rui's crate, our clothes and other light-weight items.

Diana was the first driver, and I was just noticing the problem immediately before other drivers on the sixteen lane 401 highway started honking and gesturing wildly at us. Leaning forward, I could just see the front lid of the sky-coffin was opening wider and wider. By the time Diana had managed to navigate across six lanes of 120 km/hr traffic and pull off into the parking lot of a Keg Steakhouse, a blue tarp was hanging out, and neither of us was quite sure what we'd lost. I refastened the lid, though it opened again before we got to the nearest Canadian Tire store, Plan B for all Canadian travellers' disasters. We had driven 40 km on our trip to Gaspé, with another 1400 ahead, and the start had been discouraging.

I emerged from Canadian Tire with two straps, quite similar to the Thule ones I now deeply regretted leaving at home next to our bed (it's not nearly as interesting a story as you might imagine). We tightened the new straps in place, agreed to drive at 100 km/hr to reduce the wind stress, and watched the sky-coffin closely for any intimation of further disaster. At the next stop we seared the straps' ends, so as to stop them from further unraveling which they had started in traditional Canadian Tire fashion. Surprisingly everything worked, and despite a disturbing rocking motion there were no further dropouts from the sky-coffin.

Our main concern before the drive had been Rui. Partially that was because of a misplaced trust in the quality of the sky-coffin, but this was going to be his first drive of more than one hour since we had brought him back from the breeder. He had vomited twice onto my lap during that drive, inarguably a bad travel omen, so on this trip there was enough Gravol with me to tranquilize a moderately nervous mammoth. Rui was perfect: quiet, curious, uncomplaining throughout. When we stopped, he'd leap out and pee, when we were ready to go, he'd leap back in. The first two motels we stayed at had a "no animals" policy, but relented when I explained Rui would be in his crate when he was alone. At the third

103

motel, the young woman behind the counter didn't really know the motel's policy on animals, but looked at Rui and said he seemed fine with her. Another seduction for our boy.

And so we arrived in Le Manche d'Épée, a village of about a hundred people. Our home for the next three weeks was a five room house, rented from the Fortins, a farming couple up the road. It was outside the village itself, in a valley that extended two kilometres south from the St Lawrence river. The Gaspé guidebook informed us the St Lawrence is "a river that dreams it is an ocean", and given it has tides, salt water, and an opposite bank beyond the horizon, it seemed a justifiable dream. We were about half way along a valley which only held about seven houses and was surrounded by high mountains on the three non-river sides. Our road had almost no traffic and after a five minute walk faded into a dirt path that climbed for miles into the mountains.

We settled in, unpacked what we had left (we had only lost a small folding chair and a Therm-a-Rest in the sky-coffin debacle; it could have been much worse), and moved all the furniture around the house to get it set up the way we wanted. Then we drove 6 km east along the stunningly craggy shore to Rivière St Madelaine, our nearest big town (over 250 people). We walked along the shore, a long narrowing spit between the St Lawrence and the St Madelaine rivers; the former is over 60 km wide; the latter maybe 30 metres.

This was Rui's first encounter with salt water. The day before he had taken his first few doggy paddle strokes, and he clearly enjoyed water– which he came by genetically from both his Labrador and poodle sides. He immediately knew while that he could drink the fresh water from Madelaine, he couldn't drink the salty St Lawrence. He was fascinated with the shells with partially decomposed sea creatures inside, and really enjoyed dancing along the edge of the waves, leaping back to avoid the larger ones. It was a very calm day; the waves were no more than six inches high. Earlier we had seen warning signs along the shoreline highway showing giant waves smashing over a car. There wasn't any suggestion on the sign as to what you should do under those circumstances, though rolling up your car windows was probably a good first step, and not letting your puppy play along the shore was probably a good second one.

After his immaculate behaviour during the three days it had taken to drive to Gaspé, Rui had some troubles adjusting to life in the countryside. He'd bark furiously while staring out the windows, which was puzzling: there were no cars, no people and none of the potential threats he'd see when he looked out the living room window in Toronto. Perhaps the emptiness was what spooked him? The first few times he did this I walked him around the house to show him it was safe, but finally we had to resurrect "the Death Rattle", a jar with coins in it that we shook in response to barks, to his considerable displeasure. He also barked ferociously the first time we walked by a horse, which the horse greeted with a fine combination of mild indifference and utter serenity. In Rui's defence, it was his first horse and when we walked back past it he stayed quiet, studying it very carefully to be sure it was benign. The horse remained indifferent.

We started walking with him off leash, (a delight to all three of us), up the empty mountain roads or along the beach. He generally stayed close to us, but when we got too far ahead and called him, he'd gallop back to us. We all learned to deal with his poodle fur picking up burrs quite spectacularly (like velcro, which was invented by a Swiss engineer who was cleaning burrs off his dog). And he seemed to have adjusted well to a completely new house, without chewing on anything. From the first night on he slept peacefully in our bedroom, in his crate but with the door open. It sure seemed as though he enjoyed traveling too.

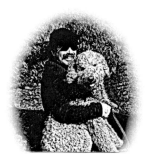

23. Gaspé Routine

"Well, all of your letters
Burned up in the fire
Time is just memory
Mixed in with desire
That's not the road; it is
Only the map.... I say
Gone, just like matches."

Tom Waits *The Part You Throw Away*

After only four days in Gaspé, we had a routine. In the morning Rui and Diana went for an early walk, with or without me. Then there would be breakfast, and a ceremony before settling into a four hour block of work: painting/drawing for Diana, writing for me. The ceremony consisted of the First Nations' pipe prayers I had been learning for about 15 years. A short summary: they are an invocation to the powers of the four directions, or mind, body, spirit, and emotion (or air, earth, fire, and water; or the animal, earth, human, and plant worlds – all archetypes have multiple manifestations.) The goal of these prayers was to define a contained sacred space separate from ordinary space. When I taught, defining a work space was easy;

I was in the classroom, and the students were in front of me. The formal school periods defined the time for work. But outside of that structure, finding a way to not be distracted (check email, play a hand of bridge, etc, etc, etc) had always been a serious challenge for me, whether the putative task was doing an essay when I was in high school, or writing a blog post, or going deeper into a problem needing a resolution. In the years since I had started doing the prayers, I had always been amazed at how they helped to bring me into the present, to bring me more fully to whatever task or issue I had focused them on. So when Diana and I planned Gaspé as a creative retreat, we had decided to try using them to carve out focused blocks of time and space for our creative work.

While we were working, Rui was outside the house, tethered to a 10 metre coated wire with its non-Rui end screwed into the ground. He liked that he could be on the porch or in our front yard; we liked that he couldn't get to the road or wander off into the unknown all around us. After work there was lunch, and then we'd all go out for an exploratory adventure.

Gaspé was a peninsula, circled by highway 132, (the one with signs warning of giant waves) and only crossed by a few roads. The part we were in, La Haut Gaspésie, (upper Gaspé) had a backbone of stark rocky mountains where few people lived. So most interior roads started as a single gravel lane quickly devolving into a path impassable by anything other than an ATV in summer, or a snow-mobile in winter. The 1:50000 topological maps we had brought with us showed many such paths, so they were the perfect guide to finding long walks without other people. Gaspé's summer weather was idyllic, sunny and crisp, about 20° C (70° F) hugely prefer-able to the smoggy swelter of Toronto. While walking, we'd pass perhaps one other person every hour, and almost no houses...just rambles across streams and through valleys lying between forested mountains.

Rui was off leash on these walks, and thus far had been perfectly behaved, sometimes hanging back to investigate interesting smells (we passed his first cow patty, which he really liked!) or stopping to pull burrs out of his paws. But he ran up to us when we called, showing no interest in leaving the path and exploring the wilderness. He loved the frequent streams and small lakes. One day we had walked for about two hours, and he was tired...the first time since early puppydom he'd been tired and I wasn't! Eventually we had come to a stream, about ten metres wide but shallow enough that he could lie down in the rocky middle with his head above water, and let the stream flow over him. This was very clearly exactly what a puppy needed at the end of a long walk, and he rested there for quite a while.

The coast had more people than the interior and some beaches were too close to the main road to let Rui run free. But others were deserted, too rocky and cold for swimming, with the only sign of human life along the shore being the occasional fishing boat. Rui loved running on sand, particularly if we were chasing him, and he'd make spectacular turns and skids to avoid the two of us. He instinctively understood pretending; if I put a fierce look in my eye and started towards him, he immediately pretended to be afraid and dodged away, whether inside or out. It was absolutely clear he knew this was a game, because he immediately became the hunter and stalked me if I started to slink away.

I thought about how all hunting animals learned to hunt by pretending with their litter mates or parents, and that all games were pretending to take seriously something that you simultaneously knew was silly. If you didn't know it was silly, it would be real not a game, and if you didn't take it seriously, you wouldn't keep doing it. Arguably if you got paid $54 million over six seasons, it stopped being a game and became serious, but Rui was clearly an amateur sports animal. He never had any trouble separating what was a game from what was real, though there were times when his divisions didn't perfectly align with ours. He once grabbed my brother's glove in –25º C. weather, and decided having everyone chasing him across a frozen lake trying to get it back was a wonderful game, despite an hour's futile attempts to convince him otherwise.

Speaking a foreign language felt like a game to me, at least partially because my limited vocabulary made me feel as though I were ten years old again. ("Oh, look. The sun is up. It will be a nice day today, will it not?") There had been a period in my teens, living in Montréal, when I could pass for French-Canadian, but four decades of neglect had weakened those skills, and now I was clearly from the separate part of the world that was English. That the Gaspégian accent is significantly different from the rest of Quebec didn't help. But while I was buying bread in the local boulangerie, my halting conversation with the baker led to my finding a house for us to rent for the two weeks at the end of the trip. It was huge (8 rooms) and by the highway so Rui couldn't play outside unattended. But it was built on a cliff over the St Lawrence so the bedroom window viewed the sun rising upstream over the river, while the dining room viewed it setting downstream. And as I sat and wrote, I could look out at whales spouting as they swam up or down. My French might be shakier than it once had been, but I'd gotten through that game.

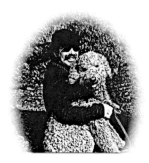

24. THE LEASH OR FREEDOM?

"And she comes to his hand
but she's not really tame
She longs to be lost
he longs for the same
and she'll bolt and she'll plunge
through the first open pass
to roll and to feed
in the sweet mountain grass"

Leonard Cohen *ballad of the absent mare*

Before we left for Gaspé, I had had a final exchange of emails with Suzanne, in which she had advised us to not let Rui off leash. Diana and I had decided we weren't going to follow her advice, because the joy of walking with Rui off leash, just the three of us meandering along, seemed greater than the danger of his wandering off. Certainly he wouldn't be outside unsupervised, to roam around at night and terrorize the Fortin's ducks, but on a walk along a remote mountain path, we didn't think much could go wrong.

Flash forward to two events in Gaspé. The first happened after we had given up on finding the walkable path that had existed when our topological maps were drawn up a decade earlier. We turned to walk back to our car just as five pick-up trucks drove by. Rui didn't want to end the walk and get back in the car, so he decided it was time to play his favourite "you can't catch me" game. He darted about the road, easily avoiding Diana and me, while the trucks slowed to a crawl to avoid this dog les maudits Anglais clearly couldn't control.

Humiliated, we finally got him back in the car and set out to find an alternative hike. We drove to a local portion of the 3500 kilometre Appalachian Trail, which either ended or started in Gaspé, depending which way you were walking. Rui hugged our legs as we walked into the bush. We came to a stream he wasn't willing to wade across. Nor would he push through the undergrowth covering the bridging logs over which we'd walked. We headed around the next bend, hoping his desire to stay with us would motivate him to cross, but all we got was the drifting sound of a piteous whimper ("Don't leave me behind!") following us. Finally Diana went back, lead him through the water, and we continued on. I warned Rui that every carnivore for miles would have heard that whimper and decided to have puppy for dinner, but he was happy enough to be with us that he ignored me.

Eventually, when we decided we weren't going to reach the mythical lake the map claimed lay somewhere ahead and we turned around to head back, Rui was suddenly transformed. He darted ahead of us, disappearing around the bends, obviously very eager to head home. We would call him, and he'd trot back, with a "Come on, let's go, what's taking you guys so long?" look on his face. But when Diana tried to grab him, he would dance away, and refuse to be touched. And each time we called him, he seemed less willing to return. Eventually we reached the stream, which he was still nervous about crossing, so we were able to leash him, and regained control.

All the puppy training books had told me the core of training a puppy is establishing I'm the alpha. The New Skete Monks cautioned about letting the dog be in charge, saying he should never be in a situation in which he decides whether he's going to come back to you or not. But I feared that was what we'd done, and while it was glorious to walk with Rui off leash, doing so left him in charge of whether he came back or not.

When we got home, we did see several black-fly bites on his belly, the only part of him that wasn't protected by his thick curly fur. Had he not been coming to us on the trail because he was so eager to get away from the flies? Black flies are insanely irritating, and I had been bothered by them on the walk, even through the miasma of DEET with which I had surrounded myself. It was the first time Rui had been bitten, so that might have been relevant. But I still thought we ought to walk him on leash from then on, even though I wanted to do otherwise. That was a hard difference to resolve. My mind said we were supposed to be in charge, and that meant we had to have our pet under control at all times. My heart wanted to accept this joyful animal into our lives as a companion, not as a chained slave, and play with him as an equal.

Rui was a microcosm of my own problem with a post–teaching career. My mind said my life should be under control, with a well-paying regular job, even if it meant I were back on a leash again. My spirit wanted to play with whichever students came to write with me in my writing course, or whatever I found online that seemed interesting enough to put in my e-magazine. I didn't have any convincing answers yet, but I certainly did admire the challenge of the problems.

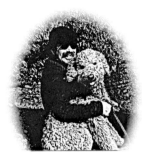

25. EXPANDING VOCABULARIES

"Drawing on my fine command of language, I said nothing."

Mark Twain

Being in a different part of Canada and speaking a different language had me thinking once again about change. When we move to another place, we need a new map and new vocabulary to navigate it. That seemed both a metaphorical and a literal truth. After leaving high school I could discard a once essential vocabulary: classes, guidelines, syllabi, rubrics. The map of my day had once been neatly compartmentalized into classes, lunch, and prep period, then so vital but now useless. My challenge after teaching could easily be seen as a struggle both to chart a new map, and find the vocabulary to navigate it.

Travelling obviously demands new maps, and new vocabularies. My earliest trip along the St. Lawrence river was in 1969 with Ceej, a close friend. We'd hitch-hiked about 50 km past Quebec City, and were still over 400 km from the ocean. Camping about 100 metres from the river one night, we woke at 3 A.M. to realize the river was only two metres from our tent, and moving in. We leapt up and moved the tent further away from the river. "Tides" hadn't been a part of our river vocabulary, but we learned it quickly. If you camp by the St Lawrence, it is an essential word.

One of the aspects of returning to Québec that I most loved was re-immersing myself in the French language and culture. That was true even if every time it seemed there was slightly less vocabulary leaping to my tongue. And while my French grammar came out like my English – I didn't think about it, it just happened – I did get a feeling what was happening had mutated considerably from the basic linguistic DNA passed on to me by one particular teacher.

Mr. Fish, whose booming, "Pierre, you nasty boy!" has haunted me these forty years, was a passionately tyrannical French teacher, to whose class I was sentenced for three of my four years in Montreal's Mount Royal High School. But while the teacher was still clear in my mind, his teachings were fading. For a return to La Belle Province it was clearly time to recharge my linguistic arsenal. I picked up a Larousse French-English dictionary for a dollar at a yard sale, but it felt so twentieth century I just had to download Ultralingua, a fine Macintosh program that lets me click on a word, press a single key, and instantly get the translation (1. traduction n.f. 2. interprétation n.f etc). When in doubt, buy a new toy....

But I hadn't fully anticipated the kind of words I'd need. Vomit, diarrhea, wart, and veterinarian weren't part of what either Mr. Fish or I had once anticipated, though Ultralingual proved adequate to the challenge. (It even conjugates verbs— "Je vomis, tu vomis, il vomit, nous vomissons .....") Rui, such a healthy dog in general, had a rough week of it. Two days after arrival we noticed a wart on his lower left lip, which went on enlarging and was joined by matching ones on his right. Diana and I observed, debating earnestly each day whether they were larger. More seriously, he suddenly stopped eating for three days, had copious diarrhea, and vomited the few times he did try to eat. Some sort of stomach bug, Diana and I agreed, though we had no way of knowing the cause. My theory was that his romps leash-free on the beach, chewing on half-rotten sea creatures in their drying out shells might be to blame; Diana wouldn't even speculate. But unambiguously, something in Québec had made him a very sick pup.

The problem was complicated not only by being in Gaspé, where we didn't have the same network of veterinary support and internet access as at home, but by it being St Jean Baptiste day, the national holiday of Québec. Directly opposite Christmas on a circular calendar, June 25th is the date Roman Catholicism chose to celebrate the birthday of John the Baptist, Jesus' cousin and harbinger. (June 25th also provided early Christians with a way to co-opt the Pagan summer solstice celebrations just as conveniently as Christmas did the winter.) But culturally, St Jean Baptiste has become a national day of celebration for all who aspire to see Québec a nation. That meant everything was closed.

Fortunately, Rui passed out the bug as the weekend passed, and by Tuesday he was eating with his usual enthusiasm, and the diarrhea had stopped. The warts were still there, but they seemed less urgent after a visit to a nearby internet café reassured us such growths are common on young dogs. Diana and I started affectionately calling him "croc des verreux"(wart fang); one of the minor joys of living with a dog is that they won't be offended by anything you say to them.

Stomach bugs weren't Rui's only new fauna; he also encountered his first rabbits. Twice we were out walking, when a rabbit came hopping down the trail towards him. Diana and I froze, and dropped the leash to see what Rui would do. He stood and watched them hop, and about thirty seconds after they'd left, carefully went forward to where they'd turned off the trail and sniffed around, as though trying to figure them out. But no hunting instinct kicked in at all... perhaps, being of retriever stock, he expected us to shoot them first, and then he'd go and retrieve them. Or perhaps he too has to learn the new vocabulary of the countryside, and the seashore and woodland creatures inhabiting it, but without a computerized downloadable dictionary to help him out on the conjugations.

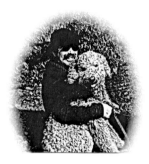

26. LEARNING TO SWIM

"This summer I went swimming
This summer I might have drowned
But I held my breath and I kicked my feet
And I moved my arms around
I moved my arms around."

Kate McGarrigle *Swimming Song*

R ui definitely hadn't gotten the natural world vocabulary down yet. On a morning walk I was barely a hundred metres from the Fortin farmhouse when we came across his first deer. Despite my best efforts to direct his attention, he remained totally focused on a stick he was chewing, and ignored the doe, who was within twenty metres. Unlike Rui, I knew what to do with nature and took photographs of it. Having satisfied one of us, the doe then wandered off, as Rui chewed on.

For the afternoon's adventure, we set off to explore the road which our topographic map showed winding for miles parallel to the Madelaine River, up into the forests and mountains to the south of us. And it may well have done so but we were never to know, as the map had failed to warn of the locked gate blocking the road barely a kilometre off the main highway. So we opted for plan B, exploring further along the kilometre of spiral spit holding the Madelaine river separate from the St Lawrence river, till it ended with their confluence.

It was a lovely sunny afternoon, maybe 20° with a mild breeze, as we walked along the much wider beach on the St Lawrence side, finding intricately marbled black and white stones (Peter and Diana) or happily gobbling more starfish (Rui). Rui ran through the salt water playing in the small waves. He was still mildly suspicious of them, and would leap out when a large one broke over his legs. Eventually we reached the end of the spit, and walked back on the Madelaine side. Rui was much more enthusiastic about fresh water, and waded into it for a serious soak and drink. While he had swum his first few strokes on a river walk we'd taken on the drive to Gaspé, he had never swum very far, or very deep, and I thought trying to lure him in was a good idea. We'd been throwing sticks for him on the beach, so I now threw one into shallow water, which he happily waded out to and brought back. (He won't drop them, but will let himself lose a tug-of-war to me so I can throw the stick again.) The next time, I threw it further, so it floated about four feet further out than the depth to which he could wade.

This was a problem! He waded in as deep as he could, and went up and down looking at the stick floating out of reach. He whimpered, but that didn't seem to change anything. Then he went a bit deeper, out of his depth, and swam parallel to the shore for a few feet, and back to where he could stand. Discovering this new method of travelling worked and could be trusted, he turned and resolutely swam out to the stick, grabbed it in his jaws, and swum back to the shore to the sound of thunderous applause from both his Alphas. He immediately showed another innate doggy instinct by running up to us and shaking himself dry when he was as close as possible.

He was clearly proud of his swimming achievement, tossing the stick in the air, catching it, and running around with it for quite a long time. Then he suddenly spotted another stick in the water and went into the river, swimming out to grab it. But he was holding his head high out of the water, which meant his paws were splashing as he paddled and pushed the stick away every time he neared it. Eventually he solved this problem and grabbed it, turned, and brought it back to the shore. Rui clearly enjoyed this new sport, racing in again when I cruelly tossed a rock in the water, even if much swimming didn't allow him to find it.

We headed back along the sea-side beach, and kept him out of the salt-water, so he wouldn't need to be washed later on. He didn't protest this, as his swimming preference was clearly waveless fresh-water, and seemed satisfied with finding further starfish on the beach. I mused on how we learn new skills when our desire pulls us out of our comfort zone. If I hadn't thrown the stick in the water, Rui probably wouldn't have gone in further than he could wade. Leaving the world of high school was my throwing my stick into water over my head, and now I had to learn to swim. Or I would learn soon... this day was sunny and warm, and didn't need anything other than what it had.

At home Rui was tired and didn't eat any supper, contenting himself with gnawing on his bone, while we dined on a marvellous lemony soufflé Diana made with tiny fresh shrimp and my salad studded with home made thyme-garlic croutons and almonds. We finished off a fine bottle of Italian red, while Rui went to sleep on our bedroom floor, onto which he vomited a large pile of half-digested starfish around six a.m. the next morning. But he did have a fine appetite for a breakfast of kibble and yogurt after a walk with Diana, and the floor is linoleum, so there was no permanent harm done. Except of course from the perspective of the starfish and the shrimp, but that was just life on the bottom links of the food chain, wasn't it?

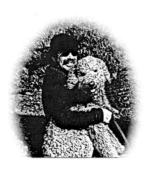

27. The Epiphany

*"If they can get you asking the wrong questions,
they don't have to worry about the answers."*

Thomas Pynchon, *Gravity's Rainbow*, "Proverbs For Paranoids"

Our Gaspé topological maps were very useful, except for the times when they weren't. But even after an incident like the locked gate, I relied on them the next time we set out for a walk. They may not have been perfect, but they were what we had. The fallible cartography reminded me of "Life And How To Survive It" a wise book written by ex-Python John Cleese together with his therapist, Dr Robyn Skynner. The book's central metaphor was that we navigated our lives with our inaccurate mental maps of the world. It argued the key distinction between successful people and the unsuccessful was the former adjusted their maps when they didn't work, and the latter just plunged on deeper into the swamps.

I thought about maps and about Rui and the map of the land of Dogdom by which I had been navigating. That was when the penny finally dropped. My map was wrong. It had alphas and betas, dominants and submissives, as the opposing continents. That was the map I had been using to understand Rui's "Muttster Hyde" behaviour, those moments when he suddenly leapt at us and bit at our hands and arms. The map had said he was a dominant when he should have been a submissive. So for the last eight months it was the core reason I had kept worrying about whether Rui was a 'Bad Dog', despite all the evidence to the contrary.

I finally realized how I'd been navigating by the wrong map. Rui was just trying to initiate a chasing game where we chase him or he chases one of us. His leaping and nipping was still an unacceptable behaviour, absolutely, but it was caused by enthusiasm, not hostility. And understanding his intent made so much difference! Diana and I could now respond without anger. I suspected just as we interpreted Rui's playfulness as anger, he had interpreted our anger as playfulness. We would grab at the leash; he would leap away; it was clearly a game. When we stopped grabbing or yelling at him, and instead just stood there and said, "Rui, down," he went from Muttster Hyde back into Doggy Jekyll with nary a whimper.

Like many insights, this was blindingly obvious in retrospect. Rui clearly wanted to play with me much of the time. When Diana, Rui, and I were walking on the Gaspé beach, Rui would often drag pieces of driftwood. Once when I was feeling playful, I picked up a heavy two meter stick and waved it over his head. "See, Rui? I can carry the biggest stick of all!" And I stuck it in the sand and looked at him. He stared back, then attacked the stick, tore it out of the sand, and proudly dragged it for ten minutes. To get him to carry an abandoned four litre milk jug we found on the beach, all I had to do was to convince him I wanted it, by playing tug-of-war with him. He carried that jug all the way back after that, past fish guts and dead seagulls. When we were nearly home, he abandoned it for black plastic tubing that flexed in an irresistible way when he bit into it. No seagulls or fish, just jugs and plastic tubing: Rui is a very urban dog.

Just as Suzanne's observation that Rui was mature for his age allowed me to recognize a whole series of mature behaviours, realizing he wanted to play let me see more of who this individual dog really was, rather than trying to fit him onto my map of abstract ideas about how dogs were in general. "How do I get Rui not to attack me?" had been the wrong question, which is why none of the answers had ever solved the problem.

And my need to be seen by others only exacerbated the problem. The primary trigger for my temper had always been being ignored, whether it was a student ignoring my repeated instructions, or a course I had shaped being redesigned by school administration without my input, or everyone deciding to head right after I'd just explained why it made much more sense to go left. I might even get set off if I thought a puppy was attacking me. And because I was so vulnerable to that feeling, I sometimes felt ignored when that wasn't the case. Recognizing the puppy just wanted to play was a big help for both of us.

Once I started to question maps, other versions of my stories became possible. Why was I unhappy with my post high school life? Because I wanted it to be like my high school life, with lots of immediate positive feedback, and a high salary. That was a perfectly good map I'd developed over thirty years but it was a Kansas map, and we weren't in Kansas any more. When I looked at my present situation – lots of creative exciting work– and enough money from my pension, I realized the extent to which the only problem was my perception there was a problem.

Had I realized six months ago that Rui's leaping and biting wasn't aggression I had to fight, how much energy would I have saved? Understanding his behaviour wasn't "bad", but well intentioned however inappropriate was a huge shift. As Hamlet said, "There's nothing neither good nor bad, but thinking makes it so." Once again, the bard had nailed it.

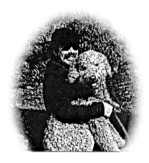

28. LEAVING GASPÉ

"And it's hey, hey. hey for the open road again
As we roll along the lonely metric miles
And it's, hey, home is anyplace she's never been
And she'll be home in just a little while"

Steve Goodman *God Bless Our Mobile Home*

As we reached the end of our five weeks in Gaspé, I thought about what the experience must have been like for Rui. I had simply assumed it would be wonderful for him to be out in the wild, because he's an animal and nature is what animals like. But of course he's very domesticated, generations removed from any ancestors who could survive in a wilderness. And it certainly wasn't our goal to have him revert to a feral state, given he was going back to Toronto, where knowing how to heel and not leaping on strangers were important, to us if not to him.

The two best aspects of those five weeks for Rui must have been the hours of off leash walks, and spending all day, every day, with both of us. The remoteness of Gaspé made off leash walks possible. We would either ramble unleashed along the sea shore, where the cliffs on one side and the sea on the other reduced his range to ahead of or behind us, or along forest paths where the thick bush did the same.

There were no people for him to leap up on, and he was increasingly happy to follow or lead, staying close to us and generally returning immediately when called. But while Diana and I delighted in the natural beauty around us, Rui was pretty indifferent. I thought of how when camping with Sam, hoping he'd learn to love nature and wilderness, I sometimes got annoyed he just wanted to play with his gameboy. Rui seemed to prefer playing with his squeaky ball, and having Diana or I throw it so he could retrieve it to investigating nature. One day our pack was on a walk when a chipmunk raced across our path. Rui showed the first predatory instinct we'd seen by dashing after it. But he kept the squeaky ball in his mouth, so we weren't sure what was going to happen if he had caught up to the chipmunk.

But I never did discern any preference in Rui for wilderness over city. Perhaps he was just a natural Buddhist taking complete joy in wherever he was. If we could have gone for long city walks and it were somehow safe for him to run freely off leash there, would he have missed being out in nature? My guess was no. Certainly in the summer he loved water, and waded into any he found, from mud puddle to sea. He was nervous about big waves (smart dog!), but small rivers clearly delighted him, and lakes were the best for swimming. But we had streams and ponds in High Park, and I suspected (correctly, as it developed) he'd be happy to go into them. Slowly I began to appreciate one of the great lessons animals teach us, the art of being in the present moment.

Rui did miss playing with other dogs, just as we missed our communities. He tried to play with country dogs, unsuccessfully. Maybe they all spoke French, and there was a communication issue? More likely, as country dogs don't have dog parks the way their city counterparts do, they don't develop doggy socialization. And of course, farm dogs are often workers, as opposed to Peter's pampered pet. The difference between these two types of dogs seemed a bit like the difference between home-schooled and public-schooled children. A country dog grows up with its owners, and whatever other dogs live there, and learns from and identifies with that pack. They've never learned the skill of socializing with strangers. My guess was that most farmers preferred it that way; large packs of dogs roaming happily across the farms would just be imminent trouble.

Home-schooled children learn from their parents and with their siblings. I had those types of students when they had transferred to high school for more advanced maths and sciences courses, and there was often a period of adjustment while they learned not to be the centre of attention, and to get along with people who were different from their family. City dogs needed to learn to get along with other dogs whom they passed on the street, or encountered in the adjacent back yard; country dogs didn't and weren't going to start with Rui.

Rui certainly loved being around Diana and I all the time. While he spent the morning (while we worked) napping, if I changed rooms he'd follow me to sleep in the new spot. When we watched videos in the evenings he'd lie down next to us, as he did during morning prayers; I called him our "dog soldier", only half in jest. And spending so much time with him allowed us to enjoy the present moments, rather than constantly worry about his training. He had become an (occasionally challenging) companion, rather just than a Good Canine Citizen in progress.

Over the summer Rui had reached his full growth, which showed up in improved coordination. He was no longer a clumsy bump–into–things puppy, but a remarkably agile beast. We saw that most on the beach, where Diana and I slowly and gingerly picked our middle–aged way over seaweed–slippery rocks, and flinty shale, while Rui rushed impeccably over them, never slipping or falling. His chest had filled out, so his growls and barks sounded deep and menacing, as we heard when the dog barked across the road or someone walked past our house.

He was spectacularly well toilet trained, as he proved on a trip to town. We'd left Rui in the car for about 90 minutes while we shopped for the week's groceries. The windows were open and he had water, not that it was terribly hot. When we got in the car and started to drive home, Rui made an intense weird moaning sound we'd never heard before. We pulled over and let him out, at which point he let loose with a spectacular bout of diarrhea. But he had waited till we let him out of the car, which was behaviour we really, really appreciated.

The hardest time we had with him was in Forillion, the stunningly gorgeous national park at the Eastern tip of Gaspé. There were three reasons he had to be leashed there: it was a rule, there were many other people on whom he was eager to leap, and there were both porcupines and mother bears with cubs around. (We saw the former, others the latter.) Rui was clearly unhappy being on a leash in wilderness and pulled enough that our three hour tug-and-walk would have been more fun without him. But when we went to Cap Ami, a nearby rocky beach, the on-call naturalist there played with Rui, then looked at us and said, "Magnifique! Il est magnifique!" And that made it all seem worthwhile.

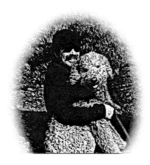

29. Beneath the Surface

"So come on in
It ain't no sin
Take off your skin
And dance around in your bones"

Tom Waits *The Black Rider*

While Rui's thick coat had been fine for ocean-cooled Gaspé, back in the humid swelter of a Toronto August his woollen poodle curls left him over-dressed, gasping in his long pants. The cost of having a non–shedding dog gets paid to the groomers. Hair grows, and it has to come off somehow. So our lamb went off to be shorn and a few hours later I picked up what looked like a totally different Rui from the one I had dropped off.

This version seemed much more intense, and alert. He definitely looked taller, due to the ratio of longer legs to a smaller torso. He engaged more with me, possibly because I could really see his eyes, rather than just catching glimpses of them. He looked like an adult dog, rather than the cross between a teddy bear and a lamb he had resembled earlier. He also panted a lot less, and had more energy for running around outside; those might have been objectively verifiable changes rather than merely reflective of my superficiality, judging by beauty when it was only skin-deep. Of course in people "skin-deep" means their outside layer, whereas Rui's skin had been hidden a long way below the furry surface.

I wondered what layers I still had to shed that were using my energy and slowing me down. My belief Rui had a Muttster Hyde inside him, a bad dog who had to be eliminated lest he take over the good doggy Jekyll, had been shed in Gaspé. Like his overly long summer fur, life had become more comfortable without it. Similarly, learning to live with Rui had involved letting go of my preconceptions about dogs. Being more fully present with the dog he really was and letting go of the fuzzy ideas I'd read might have been my equivalent to being groomed.

It had taken me many years to shed the belief I had when I had started teaching English that every grammar mistake in a student's essay had to be noted, preferably in red. I had been amazed how much more energy there was in both my students and myself once it was gone. Creating a new career after teaching was in part a process of letting go of layers of preconception over what that career would be, so I could be more aware of the actual possibilities the world was offering. One of those possibilities was The Writers' Croft. I had learned how to mentor writers in high school, and doing it online allowed me to continue with parts of what I had loved, without having to reduce the sometimes magical complexity of how someone shared their creativity to the brutal simplicity of a number that would fit in the square on the form. I advertised the September Croft and amazingly, people signed up for it.

Rui's skin wasn't the only part of him hidden from me, and I was given hints of those other parts by Elizabeth Marshall Thomas' "The Hidden Life of Dogs". She wrote the book to summarize her conclusions after over thirty years of observing the lives of the eleven dogs with whom she lived, and in whose lives she interfered as little as possible. The dogs wandered freely off leash (through Boston!), established a hierarchy, trained their young, and lived individual lives that Thomas, an anthropologist by training, observed minutely and analyzed intensely. Most of the dogs Thomas described were huskies, and her work showed the deep similarities between them and the wolves of Baffin Island she had observed when she spent time up there.

It had been a hot and muggy day, so I lay downstairs in the cooler basement, curled up next to Rui, reading the book. From time to time I stopped reading and petted him, waking him once when he started whimpering from an unhappy dream. I wondered about how much of Rui's deep essence was the same as the wolves, and about how unnatural the life we had created for him was. He doesn't live with any other dogs – instead Diana and I defined ourselves as his pack. Misha, one of the huskies Thomas described, roamed at night over 130 square miles of Boston, while Thomas rode her bike or walked behind, observing but not controlling the dog's travels. Rui was limited to brief walks mostly under our control, and always under our direction. Just as the groomer cut off Rui's fur, letting me see the actual dog beneath, so Thomas' book cut away much of the human socialization, letting me see the lupine heritage behind the domestication.

After I finished the book, Rui and I went out into the back yard. It was dark now and the humid 35° heat had let up, making the outside more pleasant. I lay back in a reclining chair and Rui crouched down a few feet away. I watched as he studied our neighbour watering plants and weeding. Then he looked away from her, keeping his head up, weaving back and forth as he analyzed the scents the breeze was bringing him. In Gaspé, Diana and I had joked about his lack of appreciation for the beautiful scenery, but of course the word "scenery" refers to what is seen. Rui appreciates the scentery, a world we are far less able to perceive, let alone appreciate, than he is the visual world. We stayed there awhile, he involved in the immediacy of the story he was distilling from the night air and I musing on the story I had just finished reading. And then we went inside and upstairs to the pack's bedroom, where Rui slept happily with his muzzle over the air-conditioning vent, something of which I was sure the wolves of Baffin Island would never have dreamed.

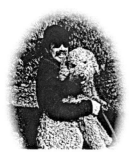

30. Intimations of Mortality

"Shadows are falling and I've been here all day
It's too hot to sleep time is running away
Feel like my soul has turned into steel
I've still got the scars that the sun didn't heal
There's not even room enough to be anywhere
It's not dark yet, but it's getting there."

Bob Dylan *It's Not Dark Yet*

If our time in Gaspé had been solid time, a continuity of intent and action weaving the days seamlessly into each other, then the four weeks following was broken time, crossed shards of purpose splintering and falling to the ground, where they lay like the bastard children of a liaison between a mosaic and a kaleidoscope. Two weeks back in Toronto catching up on the obligatory accumulations of a six week absence. Eight days in Vancouver, where my family reunion was held that year, though we also spent time with some of Diana's family when they came up from Washington State to meet us. Then back in Toronto trying to braid the missed summer past with the planned autumnal future, rarely stopping to be in the present.

And Rui, a few weeks shy of being a year old, moved through all this as a dog does, utterly in the moment. He certainly had enjoyed returning home; the moment he got into the house he ran over to his toy box, and started pulling out all the toys and old bones he hadn't seen for six weeks. When we went to Vancouver we left him with Phillipa, a dog boarder. Rui was ecstatically happy to see us when we picked him up, but as he was just as happy to greet complete strangers who came to the door, I couldn't conclude too much from that. Phillipa said he had been fine without us, but both Diana and I were struck at how much we had missed him. In "Animals in Translation", Temple Grandin said that petting a dog makes the owners happier by releasing endorphins, so perhaps it was that rush that we were missing.

Being away from him might have made the changes stand out more, but Rui had become a very different dog from the one he had been three months ago, before Gaspé. He understood the division between what he could and couldn't chew and rarely bit at our hands. He was much more obedient and docile. While certainly still playful, he would ignore some dogs, lie down peacefully when I told him to, and not engage with people on the street unless they approached him. On some walks I rarely had to pull hard or fight him, unless he saw something that might have once been food on the ground. Before the summer, walks were sometimes a continuous battle between us. These were all qualities we had been working towards. At times it seemed miraculous he was actually becoming a well trained dog.

I don't want to overstate our success: Rui wasn't fully trained. He always greeted people by leaping on them. And he still chose whether to come when called. But those were the only two major problems left. The house had its carpets back down, and the child-proof hinges were off the kitchen cupboards. Rui could roam freely and nothing got destroyed. When I said "No", he'd stop whatever he was doing. If I were writing and he brought me his ball to toss, and I just took him into the kitchen and said, once, "Rui. Kitchen. Wait." And then he would lie in the kitchen, patiently waiting to be released. I remember seeing students who as Grade Niners rushed around the classroom like puppies. And even though I kept telling them they had to learn to sit still and behave like high school students, there was a certain sadness when they did exactly that.

He was still a very playful dog and loved to be given stuffed animals so he could tear them apart, preferably with help from Diana or me. He'd bring the toy to us, so we could hold one end of it, while he'd tear ferociously at the other. When a limb came off, he'd pounce on it to pull out the exposed stuffing. Diana once took a photo of a pack of wolves tearing apart a deer carcass in a very similar way, though fluff came off the carpet more easily than blood would have. It was clear that Rui, focused and fierce in his determination to shred the toy, saw it as prey. And he retained his perennial obsession with squeaky toys, which he'd bite and chew for however long it took to destroy their squeaking ability. Perhaps the sound triggered some inherited sense of captured prey. He loved to toss the squeaky toy in the air, so it bounced away from him, and then pounce fiercely onto it. Diana and I were able to sleep more securely, knowing that should our house ever be invaded by an army of sentient squeaky toys, Rui would have the matter well in mouth.

Whether with people or other dogs, Rui's favourite game was being chased. He'd happily spend hours running away from Diana or me in the house, or yard, if we pretended to be a monster chasing him. If I stared with a particular look, and started taking Jabberwocky-sized steps towards him, he'd run and hide under the table, and dodge to another room as I reached out to grab him. But if I fled, he'd instantly turn and be in hot pursuit. Prey or predator, he understood the rules of the game. But when I put the leash on and walked him home, he'd carry the prey, squeaky or stick, as proudly in his jaws as any father wolf returning successfully from the hunt.

Benjamin Franklin once said, "We do not stop playing because we grow old. We grow old because we stop playing." Rui kept us younger too, as anyone watching two middle-aged people yelling and chasing their dog around the furniture might infer. (Either that or they'd decide we'd gone completely mad.) He had become a companion to Diana and me, and it was a rare day when he didn't make us laugh.

We had once worried about how long he would remain a puppy, and whether we could last until then. And of course maturation is always a process, not a sudden binary shift. But just as Rui looked mostly like a poodle, with a few Labrador traits, so he had become mostly dog with a few puppy traits. The saddening part was just how fast his life was passing. We had gotten him ten months earlier, and – suddenly – he was a dog, not a puppy. There was a particular flavour of energy he once had that he didn't have any more and never would again. I was rarely conscious of aging in myself; I grudgingly accepted it, that I had less hair, couldn't run as fast as I once had, but awareness of the process was elusive. (The word "denial" might have been appropriate.) That's why seeing Rui change in front of my eyes was scary. It reminded me I was perhaps making my last career choices, that any roads not taken now were probably roads I would never have the chance to take. Rui was moving towards his death, as of course we all are. As he became a better companion, I was reminded how briefly he'd be with us, and how briefly we all were to be with each other.

Rui of course didn't think about any of this. The blessing and the curse of his awareness was to always be in the present. He would lie in the kitchen while I wrote, waiting to be released from his boundary when I was finished. But the boundary of mortality, the boundary with which his maturity now confronted me, was a boundary from which there would be only one final release for either of us.

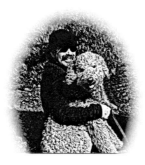

31. Reading the Subtext

"Is this the real life?
Is this just fantasy?
Caught in a landslide
No escape from reality
Open your eyes
Look up to the skies and see..."

Queen *Bohemian Rhapsody*

So, csn ynu riod tkes? And the answer for most people is yes, they can read this– the first and the last letter of each word are right, and the ascenders and descenders are in place, so we know by the shape of the word what it should be, and we leap to the meaning, as fast as Rui leapt on a visitor coming through the front door. That's why, after thinking for six months about what might be an amusing sign to alert people we had a dog, I settled for "Grand Dog on Duty", with a photo from Gaspé of Rui's leaping in the air. Over two-thirds of the people who have seen it read "Guard Dog on Duty" – that's what they expected, and what the shape of the word suggested.

That's half-way to apophenia, the tendency to see patterns where none exist. In "Blink", Malcolm Gladwell wrote about students asked to rate teachers after watching them for only 15 seconds, and the staggeringly high correlation between those ratings and those of students who'd had the same teachers for a whole semester. We glimpse the shape of a word, the style of a teacher, the tip of the iceberg and leap to a perception of what's there. We're good at recognizing familiar patterns, even when they aren't there.

Every day I walked Rui at least once, trying to understand the pattern of our relationship. And after a year of doing this, I wasn't always sure just how much I was projecting, anthropomorphizing my own emotions onto his behaviour. Generally I thought everything was coming along just fine; sometimes I thought I was spoiling him with my indulgences.

We walked on city streets, or in dog parks. Rui was always leashed on a 10 meter lead in the city. I walked the sidewalk at a constant pace while he explored the lawns and trees that lay on its safe side, as opposed to the cars and the street that lay on its suicide. Occasionally he'd tug but usually we accommodated each other. When he saw something he thought might be good to eat, a wide category, we'd have a tug of war. I'd wait for him when he had a pee; he waited for me when I retied my shoe. When I said, "Heel", Rui would walk next to me for a few minutes. Otherwise he'd wander, exploring his world. He'd listen to my instructions, and sometimes obey them.

Some books had offered a vision of a dog as an autonomous companion creature, and I thought Rui and I were doing okay by those standards. Some (a popular TV show whispered its name) saw a dog as a subservient creature who should always do what you wanted. It made sense guide dogs for the blind should heel all the time, and not suddenly dash off after abandoned pizza. But did that make sense for Rui?

I didn't know. The problem was I wanted him to choose to trot alongside me, and to always come back when was called, to be a companion rather than a slave. I wanted Rui to be an independent dog, who chose of his own volition to do exactly as he was told. I recognized the problem with this position, which was akin to Israel saying they wanted Palestine to be a free democracy, as long as they never voted for Hamas. Looking at those things I didn't like in Rui's behaviour, it seemed unsure if he'd grow out of them, (as he had with inappropriate chewing.) Perhaps these were clear signs an intervention was needed before he became an old dog who wouldn't give up his bad tricks? Or were they just part of who he was, a blessed combination of good and bad, just as you are and I am? Was the glass half full, half empty, or merely twice as big as it needed to be?

The warning picture on our front porch appeared to show Rui leaping fiercely into the air, but that too was false. The truth was before I photoshopped myself out he was leaping playfully into my arms. Visitors too could see a loving dog and misread him as dangerous. Guard dog or grand dog? Teaching with love, or spoiling with overindulgence? Where was his training going, and where did I really want it to go? I groped blindly through this fog of uncertainty, holding tightly to one end of the leash joining Rui and me. But by now I knew that we were on this trip together, and we were both sometimes trusty guides and sometimes blind. I just hoped the pizza scraps didn't get too distracting, for either of us.

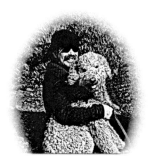

32. The Year of Living Doggedly

"I've got to admit it's getting better
A little better all the time
I have to admit it's getting better
It's getting better since you've been mine."

The Beatles *Getting Better*

It was now one year since Rui had come into our lives, or from the other end of the leash, one year since we had come into his. Last November he had been a three kilogram puppy only nine weeks old, who wriggled happily on my lap as we drove him away from his mother and the farm where he was born, and into the big city. Now he lay on my feet, a 25 kilogram dog who wriggled happily as he gnawed on an old favourite knuckle bone hoping to liberate a last shred of marrow. Rui has always been a dog who wriggled happily.

I'd learned a lot about dogs in this year, from books, dog trainers, and from surrealistically similar conversations with other dog owners in parks while we watched our animals run and romp, and took turns trotting after them clutching our little plastic bags ready to scoop. Most of all I'd learned from Rui, who was training and teaching us, as we did him. Some teachings were simple: something he really wanted to eat, such as the oily salmon skin left after dinner, might come up almost as fast as it had gone down. Desire was never a completely reliable guide to what was good, no more for him than for me.

Other lessons were more complex, the meta-teachings about teaching being the most complicated. Working with a dog, I'd concluded, had similarities to teaching teenagers: if you let them know you liked them, and consistently let them know what you wanted, it would probably all work out. I'd also learned that, as with students, each dog was different. Books on teaching, and teacher training courses were all often useful, but you had to treat the Other as a unique and specific individual. That's when the real relationships formed, and when the magic started to happen. Sometimes that meant not following instructions and trusting your heart rather than the textbook. In the Croft I was discovering the joy of teaching with no one to report to, and the gift of always being able to respond to what seemed the most important. My students valued it too; my biggest surprise in the next years of the Croft was over half of them would return to take the course repeatedly.

Rui had matured from a dog who had chewed everything he could get his teeth into; even locked in the kitchen he had managed to tear the moulding off the walls and reduce parts of it to kindling. A year later he roamed the house freely, and never chewed anything other than his toys. He still hadn't learnt to speak and almost never barked, except when he was trying to persuade a person or dog to play with him. But he had learned to communicate clearly, whether by nudging my mouse hand so I couldn't use a computer when he felt I needed to focus on him rather than on the screen, or by nudging the bell on the back door when he wanted to go out.

He was a reasonably smart dog, and usually understood what Diana and I wanted, though just as we didn't always give him what he wanted, he didn't always give us what we wanted. It was harder for him because my goals had been uncertain. He was remarkably good natured, even by doggy standards, which are far higher than human ones. At a park, Rui would go over and nuzzle all the dog owners as well (and sometimes before) he nuzzled all the other dogs. In my writing group he would get up off my feet and wander around to all the other members and nudge them, so that they'd know if they weren't interested in writing any more and wanted to play with a dog instead, he was available. And when I wrestled him and forced my hand into his mouth to pry a chicken bone out before he could choke himself on it, he never bore any grudge.

Being an animal, he was very in his body. And that made me be more in mine, particularly through giving him his two daily walks (with Diana's help) every day. That certainly had caused a more planned structure to my days than I'd had previously (no more spontaneously spending an afternoon wandering through Kensington Market) but it also meant more exercise (no more afternoons wedged before the computer). And there had been more computer afternoons than Kensington Market afternoons.

Instead of being locked in the kitchen, Rui slept in our bedroom, either at the foot of the bed or beside it, moving around spontaneously. That made midnight trips to the bathroom a bit more challenging, particularly as he had an absolute faith I wouldn't step on him. So he wouldn't move until I did step on him, an event that did not appear to shake his trust the next night. Perhaps he felt he was training me to see in the dark. Sometimes we forgot to close the door at night, so he could have gotten out and wandered through the house. But he stayed with us, obviously feeling the shared bedroom was the correct place for the pack to sleep, though he did nap in his old crate downstairs when Diana and I were in the living room. It no longer had its metal door mounted, so he lay in it with his nose out, half asleep but half alert.

My 94 year old British aunt observed, with her customary perspicacity, that Diana and I were besotted with him. And it was true that as we exchanged tales of what he had done on his morning walk, and how he had almost chased a squirrel in the park in the afternoon we sounded like puppyrazi trading tales of our favourite celebrity and his doings. But the sharing of anecdote, responsibility, and love for Rui had brought Diana and I closer. As two adults we had been one kind of household; as two adults and a dependent we were another. Of course there were simple issues such as whether she could do the Thursday morning walk, if I were out late Wednesday. But beyond that, there was the deep joy of sharing the complex and tender challenge of this creature who lived with us.

But most of all, perhaps unexpectedly, what Rui had brought to us was an affectionate and independent spirit demanding we meet him and engage. He wanted physical contact with us, and he wanted to play. He would do what we wanted him to, most of the time, but had a strong will of his own. A year into this relationship I laughed more, exercised more, and was a happier person. If I didn't know what exactly my future held, I had at least learned from Rui to wriggle happily and enjoy the present. While there were still things I hoped to teach him, I had also come to know there was a lot to learn from him.

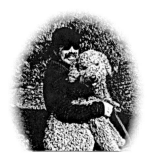

33. RUI TAKES PETER FOR A WALK

"Today, like every other day, we wake up empty
and frightened. Don't open the door to the study
and begin reading. Take down a musical instrument.

Let the beauty we love be what we do.
There are hundreds of ways to kneel and kiss the ground."

Rumi

Perhaps it was because my back had been spasming for three days, and my usual walk with Rui still involved tugging to get him not to sample some potentially tasty object, or to slow his dogtrot down to a human pace. He was an enthusiastic 25 plus kilos of labradoodle, and that day both maneuvers seemed as though they would be painful. Or perhaps it was because I had recently finished Elizabeth Marshall Thomas' "The Hidden Life of Dogs", and had been amazed at how she let her eleven dogs live alongside her without trying to direct and control their behaviour. So as we went out the door, it suddenly occurred to me to try something new, something never tried before. I'd let Rui lead the walk.

We had been living together for ten months, going out twice a day for walks, and that this was the first time I was actually going to let him choose where we would go probably says something about the extent I'm deeply in touch with my inner fascist. Like all right-wingers, I was deeply convinced it was only for Rui's good that I controlled where we went and what we did when we got there. But today was going to be different… there was time to spare, no appointments, and I was curious. He was enthusiastic, as always, about going out for a walk, and sat at the top of the porch stairs waiting for me to say it was okay to go. I nodded and gave the command, and he walked down the steps, down the pathway to the sidewalk, glanced in both directions and then looked back up at me. I looked down at him. "Your call today, pup."

He turned and headed south down Margueretta Street. As he started to head into a neighbour's house via an open front door, I realized I couldn't give him unlimited freedom. The fewest restrictions needed were no going into people's houses, no meandering out onto the street, and no eating garbage. That seemed a fair set to me, so I told Rui who as usual didn't deign to comment one way or the other.

Two interesting behaviours stood out. Rui went a lot more slowly down the street than I usually do, thoroughly exploring most of the front yards we passed. He would carefully smell things in the front yard, rarely stopping to mark territory, but not skipping anything, rather as though there was an imminent final in his "Smells of Margueretta Street" course, and he was meticulously reviewing the material. A few houses had "Beware of Dog" signs, and he was particularly interested in exploring those front yards, from which I concluded either he had learned to read, or he could smell the dogs the signs warned us of. Sometimes one of them would start fiercely barking from a backyard, or from inside the house, at which Rui would first look mildly interested but then ignore, neither barking back nor hurrying with his exploration of the other dog's territory.

The other interesting thing was the extent to which he clearly has inculcated the idea of the purpose of a walk being to go some-where. While he went more slowly, and clearly paid much more attention to where we were at any given moment in the world of scents and odours than he could have on my faster walks, he had a definite goal that lay further ahead. After exploring each yard, and leaving his mark on a few, he continued down the street neither going back towards home nor trying to cross the street.

The block on which we lived happened to be the longest in the city of Toronto. If I walked once around it, I would have gone over a mile (and even further if I were walking in metric!) So it took a while until we reached College, the first cross street, given how many interesting front yards needed to be explored. When we got there, Rui went into a small space a bit too small to even be called a parkette. It had been a pile of junk by the side of an industrial building until a year ago, when someone cleared it up, putting a grey gravel pathway leading into a centre space, with a patch of wildflowers on one side and a bench on the other. Rui immediately headed into this space and began to explore it. Sitting down on a bench, I thought about how I'd never stopped there before as I'd always been going somewhere else and passed it, and been too in-tent on getting there to stop. But I wasn't going anywhere this day, so I sat and enjoyed the tranquility of it, while Rui wriggled his way beneath the bench in a serious attempt to determine if there was anything left of whatever smelled so good. At last he sadly concluded there wasn't, and we got up and continued.

With no hesitation he turned right, and headed along College to-wards McGregor Park, two blocks west, at Lansdowne. That was our closest park, and we went there a lot as it was enclosed, so Rui could run off leash. But had he assumed that was where I wanted him to go, or did he want to go there himself? It made sense he didn't want to go back towards home, which would have meant ending the walk, but there were two other directions he might have chosen, and I was slightly surprised and intrigued while I tended to choose novelty over familiarity; Rui did not.

We got to the park, and he stood at the gate, until I opened it, and we went inside. I took his leash off, and he wandered around. Sometimes in the afternoon there were two dog walkers there, which he liked: each brought along at least ten dogs with whom he could play. But that day there was no one, so we sat beneath a tree. Eventually I said, "Rui, let's go home" and he looked at me, got up and stretched, and walked towards the gate. As we left we met a mother walking a four year old daughter. The mother was almost completely bald, with a few straggly hairs that suggested chemotherapy rather than style. We chatted, as her daughter was very interested in Rui. When I reassured her he was a friendly dog she petted him while he lay placidly at her feet which he occasionally licked, to her great delight. She was amazed he was only one year old, and happily boasted, "I'm four. I'm much older than he is."

I ended his limited freedom shortly thereafter, as it occurred to me (it may have already occurred to Rui) that if he were left making decisions we might never get home. I wasn't sure he would mind this, certainly not for a long time, but there was a spinach and tomato dhal I planned to cook before Diana got back and we'd already been out for an hour and a half. Rui seemed very agreeable to following my suggested directions, and it struck me how much we can take walks together now. A few months ago he would often have disagreed with my ideas about where to go and I'd make him follow; but now he was comfortable with my choices. And I had learnt to let him pick the pace, so he could explore and learn what he needed to about the important neighbourhood changes to which I seemed so curiously insensitive. The freedom experiment was a great success, and Rui seemed very pleased his training of me was finally working out.

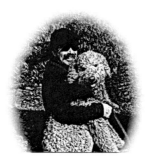

ACKNOWLEDGEMENTS

Six years ago a nine week old labradoodle puppy named Rui arrived in Diana's and my lives. I posted irregularly on my blog amusing anecdotes and such insights as I had into the experience of figuring out how to live with this strange new being. It was when Diana and I went to Gaspé, about eight months later, that I first had the idea that with a little editing those posts might form a book. Five years and four drafts later I am grateful that I had no realistic idea of quite how much work was involved. But I kept hearing two recurrent refrains from friends and editors when I showed them the work in progress: "This is really good" and "This could be even better". Oftentimes the ways they felt the manuscript could be improved were contradictory, but without all their support this book would never have been born.

Two writing groups heard both the original posts, and their revisions through the years. One is the writing group with whom I've met biweekly for almost twenty years; the other the various members of the Writers' Croft, an online writing program. Without their enthusiasm, and their surprisingly (to me, for sure) positive responses I might never have thought I had a book worth publishing. In particular, Wilder Penfield, Carolyn Hassard, and Pilar Patterson were always willing to read and responded with insight and compassion. Thanks as well to Cath, Gord, and Dave.

Mom has been a continual support throughout, both to me and to Rui, whom she calls "her canine grandchild". Oriah Mountain Dreamer has been a mentor throughout the book (and much else) and I am hugely grateful for her ongoing inspiration. Alex Schultz edited an early draft, led me up the mountain, and showed me a vision of how much better the book could be. This was both depressing (I had thought it was finished) and useful (he was right; it wasn't close). In particular, Alex first pointed out what I hadn't yet realized; the book was about my journey more than it was about Rui. Rob Starr was a delight to work with as copy editor; he consistently pared down my excess verbiage and found more solecisms than I would ever have believed could have escaped my English teacher's eye.

Most of all thanks beyond words go to Diana Meredith, whose unwavering faith and support kept me going though the book as though life. Without her, nada. While Rui was always an inspiring subject, to my regret he remains adamantly unwilling to share any thoughts about his depiction in these pages.

CPSIA information can be obtained at www.ICGtesting.com
Printed in the USA
LVOW040316270712

291561LV00001B/8/P